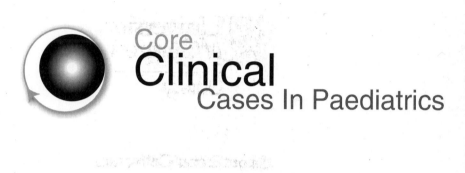

Core
Clinical
Cases In Paediatrics

Core Clinical Cases

Titles in the series include:

Core Clinical Cases in Paediatrics
Authors: Andrew Ewer, Timothy G. Barrett & Vin Diwakar

Core Clinical Cases in Psychiatry
Authors: Tom Clark, Ed Day & Emma C. Fergusson

Coming soon…

Core Clinical Cases in Basic Biomedical Science
Author: Samy Azer

Core Clinical Cases in Obstetrics & Gynaecology 2nd Edition
Authors: Janesh K. Gupta, Gary Mires & Khalid S. Khan

Core Clinical Cases in the Medical and Surgical Specialities
Edited by Steve Bain & Janesh K. Gupta

Core Clinical Cases in Medicine & Surgery
Edited by Steve Bain & Janesh K. Gupta

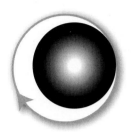

Core
Clinical
Cases In Paediatrics

A problem-solving approach

Andrew Ewer MD MRCP FRCPCH
Senior Research Fellow, University of Birmingham;
Honorary Consultant Neonatologist,
Birmingham Women's Hospital, Birmingham, UK.

Timothy Barrett PhD MRCP MRCPCH
Honorary Consultant and Senior Lecturer,
Department of Endocrinology,
Birmingham Children's Hospital, Birmingham, UK

Vin Diwakar MB BS MRCP
Consultant Paediatrician, Birmingham Children's Hospital,
Birmingham, UK

Core Clinical Cases series edited by

Janesh K. Gupta MSc MD FRCOG
Clinical Senior Lecturer/ Honorary Consultant in
Obstetrics and Gynaecology, University of Birmingham,
Birmingham Women's Hospital, Birmingham, UK

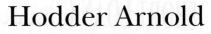

Hodder Arnold

A MEMBER OF THE HODDER HEADLINE GROUP

First published in Great Britain in 2005 by
Hodder Arnold, an imprint of Hodder Education,
an Hachette Livre UK Company,
338 Euston Road, London NW1 3BH

http://www.hoddereducation.co.uk

Whilst the advice and information in this book are believed to be true and
accurate at the date of going to press, neither the author[s] nor the publisher
can accept any legal responsibility or liability for any errors or omissions
that may be made. In particular, (but without limiting the generality of the
preceding disclaimer) every effort has been made to check drug dosages;
however it is still possible that errors have been missed. Furthermore,
dosage schedules are constantly being revised and new side-effects
recognized. For these reasons the reader is strongly urged to consult the
drug companies' printed instructions before administering any of the drugs
recommended in this book.

British Library Cataloguing in Publication Data
A catalogue record for this book is available from the British Library

Library of Congress Cataloging-in-Publication Data
A catalog record for this book is available from the Library of Congress

ISBN: 978 0 340 81668 4

3 4 5 6 7 8 9 10

Commissioning Editor: Georgina Bentliff
Project Editor: Heather Smith
Production Controller: Jane Lawrence
Cover Design: Georgina Hewitt
Index: Indexing Specialists (UK) Ltd

Typeset in 9 on 12 pt Frutiger Light Condensed by Phoenix Photosetting, Chatham, Kent
Printed and bound in Malta

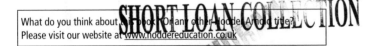

What do you think about this book? Or any other Hodder Arnold title?
Please visit our website at www.hoddereducation.co.uk

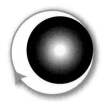

Contents

We would like to thank Rachel, Emma and Kate without whose constant support this book would not have been written. We would also like to thank Ellen, Sophie, Alice, George, Joseph and Lydia for their wonderful drawings.

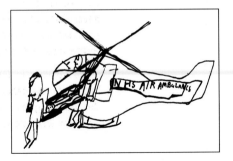

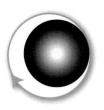

Series preface

'A History Lesson'

Between about 1916 and 1927 a puzzling illness appeared and swept around the world. Dr von Economo first described encephalitis lethargica (EL), which simply meant 'inflammation of the brain that makes you tired'. Younger people, especially women, seemed to be more vulnerable but the disease affected people of all ages. People with EL developed a 'sleep disorder', fever, headache and weakness, which led to a prolonged state of unconsciousness. The EL epidemic occurred during the same time period as the 1918 influenza pandemic, and the two outbreaks have been linked ever since in the medical literature. Some confused it with the epidemic of Spanish flu at that time while others blamed weapons used in World War I.

Encephalitis lethargica (EL) was dramatised by the film Awakenings (book written by Oliver Sacks who is an eminent Neurologist from New York), starring Robin Williams and Robert De Niro. Professor Sacks treated his patients with L-dopa, which temporarily awoke his patients giving rise to the belief that the condition was related to Parkinson's disease.

Since the 1916-1927 epidemic, only sporadic cases have been described. Pathological studies have revealed an encephalitis of the midbrain and basal ganglia, with lymphocyte (predominantly plasma cell) infiltration. Recent examination of archived EL brain material has failed to demonstrate influenza RNA, adding to the evidence that EL was not an invasive influenza encephalitis. Further investigations found no evidence of viral encephalitis or other recognised causes of rapid-onset parkinsonism. MRI of the brain was normal in 60% but showed inflammatory changes localised to the deep grey matter in 40% of patients.

As late as the end of the 20th century, it seemed that the possible answers lay in the clinical presentation of the patients in the 1916-1927 epidemic. It had been noted by the clinicians at that time that the CNS disorder had presented with pharyngitis. This led to the possibility of a post-infectious autoimmune CNS disorder similar to Sydenham's chorea, in which group A beta-hemolytic streptococcal antibodies cross-react with the basal ganglia and result in abnormal behaviour and involuntary movements. Anti-streptolysin-O titres have subsequently been found to be elevated in the majority of these patients. It seemed possible that autoimmune antibodies may cause remitting parkinsonian signs subsequent to streptococcal tonsillitis as part of the spectrum of post-streptococcal CNS disease.

Could it be that the 80-year mystery of EL has been solved relying on the patient's clinical history of presentation, rather than focusing on expensive investigations? More research in this area will give us the definitive answer. This scenario is not dissimilar to the controversy about the idea that streptococcal infections were aetiologically related to rheumatic fever.

With this example of a truly fascinating history lesson, we hope that you will endeavour to use the patient's clinical history as your most powerful diagnostic tool to make the correct diagnosis. If you do you are likely to be right 80 to 90% of the time. This is the basis of all the Core Clinical Cases series, which will make you systematically explore clinical problems through the clinical history of presentation, followed by examination and then the performance of appropriate investigations. Never break that rule.

Janesh Gupta
2005

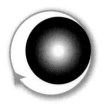

Foreword

As a paediatric student nearly 40 years ago, I went onto the children's ward of my Teaching Hospital for the first time, and picked up a small green textbook, which was mainly a series of lists. It helpfully enumerated – without description – 200 causes of abdominal pain in children, 150 causes of failure to thrive, and over 100 causes of short stature. Could this be what paediatrics was going to be about? Fortunately not. Thankfully, fashions in clinical education have changed, and books of lists are no more.

This book represents a much more relevant, context-based approach to teaching paediatrics and child health, and is one that has proven popular with students in Birmingham over a number of years. Paediatric symptoms from infancy and childhood are presented, followed by a practical approach to solving them. They have been assembled by a small, expert group of authors and chosen carefully, because they are important – either because they are frequent, or because the symptom may indicate a serious or dangerous underlying disorder. The content is relevant to both undergraduate medical students and to postgraduates and probably to nurses in training too. It is not comprehensive – were it to be, its point would be lost.

I am delighted to be able to commend this book to you. It contains a distillate of the authors' clinical acumen and wisdom. Consequently, there is hardly a list in sight.

Professor Ian Booth
Leonard Parsons Professor of Paediatrics and Child Health
The Medical School
Edgbaston
Birmingham
UK

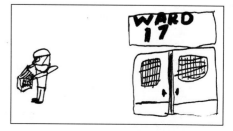

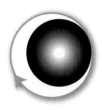

Abbreviations

ADH	antidiuretic hormone
ALT	alanine aminotransferase
ASO	anti-streptolysin O
AST	aspartate aminotransferase
CMV	cytomegalovirus
DAT	direct antibody test
ESR	erythrocyte sedimentation rate
FBC	full blood count
FSH	follicle-stimulating hormone
γ-GT	γ-glutamyl transferase
G-6PD	glucose 6-phosphate dehydrogenase
GNRH	gonadotrophin-releasing hormone
HSP	Henoch–Schönlein purpura.
IGF	insulin-like growth factor
ITP	idiopathic thrombocytopenic purpura
ITU	intensive therapy unit
LH	luteinizing hormone
LHRH	luteinizing hormone-releasing hormone
LRTI	lower respiratory tract infection
NAI	non-accidental injury
PEFR	peak expiratory flow rate
RSV	respiratory syncytial virus
SIADH	syndrome of inappropriate ADH
TORCH	screen for Toxoplasma, Rubella, Cytomegalovirus, Herpes simplex
URTI	upper respiratory tract infection
UTI	urinary tract infection

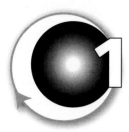

Growth problems

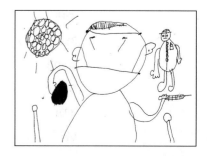

? Questions for each of the clinical cases

Q1: What is the likely differential diagnosis?
Q2: What issues in the given history support the diagnosis?
Q3: What additional features in the history would you seek to support a particular diagnosis?
Q4: What clinical examination would you perform, and why?
Q5: What investigations would be most helpful, and why?
Q6: What treatment options are appropriate?

Clinical cases

● CASE 1.1 – My 6-year-old son is the shortest in his class.

A 6-year-old boy was seen in the paediatric outpatient department. His parents complained that he was the shortest boy in his class, and he could not reach the coat pegs in school. On examination, the child's height was 106 cm (3rd centile).

● CASE 1.2 – My 5-year-old daughter is developing breasts.

A 5-year-old girl was referred to outpatients because of early breast development. This had been present since birth, but is increasing. She was on no medication. On examination, her height was 117 cm (98th centile). Breast development was Tanner stage 2.

● CASE 1.3 – My 14-year-old daughter has not yet started her periods.

A 14-year-old girl was referred for investigation of delayed puberty. She was born at full term, after a normal pregnancy. Her general development was normal, and she attended a mainstream school. On examination, she was prepubertal.

OSCE counselling cases

OSCE COUNSELLING CASE 1.1 – Can you give my son something to make him taller?

OSCE COUNSELLING CASE 1.2 – Why is my child overweight?

🔑 Key concepts

In order to work through the core clinical cases in this chapter, you will need to understand the following key concepts.

Phases of childhood growth

- Infancy phase: from birth to 2–3 years, the fastest period of growth. It is determined mainly by nutrition.

- Childhood phase: from 2–3 years to the onset of puberty, and is determined mainly by hormones, including growth hormone, thyroxine and insulin.

- Adolescent growth spurt: occurs from the onset of puberty to fusion of the epiphyses, and is determined by the synergistic action of growth hormone and sex hormones (androgens and oestrogens).

Fusion of epiphyses

A gradual process initiated by the secretion of oestrogen from the adrenals in boys and ovaries in girls. Epiphyseal fusion limits final adult height.

Precocious puberty

The development of secondary sexual characteristics before the ages of 8 years in females and 9 years in males. One example is thelarche, which is the isolated development of breast tissue without pubic or axillary hair development.

Delayed puberty

The absence of pubertal development by 14 years of age in females and 15 years in males.

Tanner staging

The classification of pubertal development according to the appearance of pubic hair in males and females, breast development in females, and external genital development in males. Stage 1 is prepubertal, stage 5 is adult.

Orchidometer

A series of beads of increasing size from 2 mL volume to 24 mL volume used to assess testicular size. Testicular volume increases in proportion to testosterone secretion. Volumes of 2–3 mL equates to prepubertal testicular size; 12 mL volume is attained at the time of maximum height velocity. From 12 mL upwards is normal for male adults.

Measurement of height and height velocity

- To determine the true height velocity, children should have their height measured on two occasions at least 6 months apart. This reduces measurement inaccuracies due to observer error. The accuracy of a single height measurement is ± 0.5 cm. Inter-observer error is similar. To minimize these errors, the height should be measured by the same person, on the same equipment, with a minimum interval of 6 months.

- The height attained over a 6-month period can be doubled to express a height velocity in cm per year. Centile charts exist for height velocity. A child's height velocity needs to remain above the 25th centile in order to maintain the centile on a linear growth chart.

- Height velocity below the 25th centile for at least 18 months equates to a child drifting down the centiles on a linear growth chart, and is one definition of growth failure.

Estimation of final adult height from parents' height (mid-parental height)

To estimate a boy's final height, add 12.5 cm to mother's height and take the mean of the mother's adjusted height and the father's height (mid-parental height). For a girl's final height, subtract 12.5 cm from the father's height and take the mean of the adjusted father's height and the mother's height. The 95 per cent confidence limits for the child's predicted adult height are the mid-parental height ± 8 cm.

Turner syndrome

- A common cause of short stature in girls, with a prevalence of about 1 in 5000. It is caused by the absence of one of the sex chromosomes, giving a karyotype of 45XO.

- Features include short stature, web neck, wide carrying angle at the elbow, convex nails, shield-shaped chest, low posterior hairline, ovarian dysgenesis (defective development), and normal intelligence (but sometimes difficulty in socialization).

- Girls with Turner syndrome are relatively growth hormone-resistant, but they do benefit from growth hormone treatment, which can increase their final height by about 5 cm.

- These girls also need hormone replacement in the form of oestrogens to induce puberty.

- Many children and parents benefit by getting in touch with a family support group such as the Child Growth Foundation.

Answers

⬤ **CASE 1.1 – My 6-year-old son is the shortest in his class.**

 Q1: What is the likely differential diagnosis?

A1

- Familial short stature.
- Constitutional delay of growth.
- Psychosocial causes of short stature.
- Isolated growth hormone deficiency.

 Q2: What issues in the given history support the diagnosis?

A2

The boy is on the third centile for height, which means that 3 per cent of the population of 6-year-olds are shorter than him. He is within the normal range of height for a UK population. Consequently, he is likely to be a short, normal boy.

 Q3: What additional features in the history would you seek to support a particular diagnosis?

A3

- Ask how long the parents have been worried, i.e. has he always been short or small; is there any history of chronic illness? (e.g. coeliac disease (q.v.), heart or kidney disease)
- Was he a normal birth and delivery? (ask about birthweight). Was he born premature or growth restricted? (constitutional short stature)
- What ethnic group is the family from? (ethnic differences in height) How tall are his parents? (familial short stature)
- What is the social background and family relationships? (emotional neglect or other forms of child abuse are causes of psychosocial short stature)
- Is he falling behind his peers? (height falling off centiles as in growth hormone deficiency)

 Q4: What clinical examination would you perform, and why?

A4

- Measure his parents' height and plot them on the growth chart.
- Estimate mid-parental height.

Q5: What investigations would be most helpful, and why?

A5

- Take serial height measurements at least 6 months apart.

- Calculate height velocity. If height velocity is below 25th centile over 6 months, other investigations would include:

  - Measurement of insulin-like growth factor-1 (IGF1) as a surrogate marker of growth hormone.

  - X-ray of the left wrist to ascertain bone age or skeletal maturity. This is delayed in growth hormone deficiency. Other causes of bone age delay include hypothyroidism and coeliac disease.

  - Growth failure is an indication for formal pituitary testing with a dynamic growth hormone stimulation test such as the insulin stress test in which a small dose of insulin is given to induce hypoglycaemia. This is a potent stimulus for growth hormone secretion, and serial measurements assess the peak secretion.

 Q6: What treatment options are appropriate?

A6

- The most likely diagnosis is familial short stature. No treatment is necessary, but reassurance that the child is normal.

- Constitutional short stature is usually not amenable to treatment, although some children with Russell Silver syndrome (a disorder of short stature, hemihypertrophy, incurved little fingers, and triangular shaped face) do benefit from growth hormone therapy.

- Psychosocial short stature will respond to elimination of the causes of emotional neglect or other forms of child abuse. This may require removal of the child from the abusing environment.

 CASE 1.2 – My 5-year-old daughter is developing breasts.

 Q1: What is the likely differential diagnosis?

A1

- Isolated thelarche.

- Thelarche variant.

- Precocious puberty.

Q2: What issues in the given history support the diagnosis?

A2

The child is not on any medication, and some breast development has been present since birth.

Q3: What additional features in the history would you seek to support a particular diagnosis?

A3

- Ask whether parents have noticed any pubic hair or unusual mood swings (precocious puberty). In addition, has the child been growing rapidly over the past 1–2 years, as in an adolescent growth spurt?

- Has anyone else in the family had early breast development? Did this progress to precocious puberty?

 Q4: What clinical examination would you perform, and why?

A4

- Plot the growth on a height and weight chart, together with previous measurements to gauge her height velocity. A rapid height velocity would suggest an adolescent growth spurt, and precocious puberty. Check mid-parental height.

- Examine for pubic and axillary hair – again, signs of precocious puberty – and perform an abdominal examination for masses.

- Consider neurological examination. Intra-cranial tumours are a rare cause of precocious puberty, more common in boys, and usually resulting in disconsonant puberty (pubic hair without testicular enlargement).

Q5: What investigations would be most helpful, and why?

A5

- If there are no other signs of puberty, then isolated premature thelarche is the most likely diagnosis. This is a benign condition, and may not require follow-up. Parents can be instructed to contact the doctor again if further signs of puberty develop.

- If the child's height is above the expected centile for the parents' height, then serial measurements of growth are required to detect a premature growth spurt. In addition, a bone age X-ray will give an indication of possible advanced bone age. If the bone age is advanced in the absence of other signs of puberty, the child fits into the category of thelarche variant. These children are at risk of developing precocious puberty, and require follow-up.

- The presence of other signs of puberty such as pubic hair, warrants further investigations. These include a pelvic ultrasound for ovarian follicles and uterine size, and a luteinizing hormone-releasing hormone (LHRH) test. An injection of LHRH is given, and luteinizing hormone (LH) and follicle-stimulating hormone (FSH) measured at time points after. The magnitude of the rise in LH and FSH indicates whether the child is prepubertal, in early puberty, or established puberty. True precocious puberty is usually of central origin at the level of the hypothalamus, and the cause is unknown.

Q6: What treatment options are appropriate?

A6

- The most likely diagnosis is isolated premature thelarche. In this situation, the parents can be reassured and the child does not need to be followed-up.

- If thelarche variant is present, the child needs follow-up as she is at risk of precocious puberty.

- If precocious puberty is present, it is important to delay further progression to avoid compromising final height, and to prevent the onset of menarche in primary school. The available treatment is depot injection of a gonadotrophin-releasing hormone agonist such as goserelin. This acts by down-regulating the release of LH and FSH from the anterior pituitary, and may regress pubertal signs.

⬤ CASE 1.3 – My 14-year-old daughter has not yet started her periods.

 Q1: What is the likely differential diagnosis?

A1

- Familial delayed puberty.

- Turner syndrome.

- Systemic illness.

- Anorexia nervosa.

Q2: What issues in the given history support the diagnosis?

A2

This girl is presumably of normal development and intelligence as she attends a mainstream school. Age at menarche has a large genetic component, and tends to run in families. However, Turner syndrome must be excluded.

 Q3: What additional features in the history would you seek to support a particular diagnosis?

A3

- Ask about mum's age at menarche, and the ages of menarche of any sisters.

- Is the girl short compared to her peers? (Turner syndrome)

- Does she have any chronic illness such as cystic fibrosis (q.v.) that would explain her delayed puberty?

- Are there any factors in the social history that would lead you to suspect anorexia (pressure of examinations, unusual fixation with food, unwillingness to develop adult interests and behaviour).

Q4: What clinical examination would you perform, and why?

A4

- Plot height and weight on a growth chart. Check the parents' height.

- Look for short stature in relation to parents' heights (Turner) and underweight for height (anorexia).

- Assess her pubertal stage. Is she prepubertal? (the commonest situation in Turner)
- Does she have hyperteleorism, web neck, wide carrying angle of the arms, shield chest, hypoplastic nails, underdeveloped nipples, or other signs of Turner syndrome?

Q5: What investigations would be most helpful, and why?
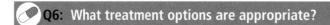

A5

- Chromosome karyotype. The normal female complement should be 46XX. Turner girls are usually mosaic (i.e. they have a mixture of cells, some normal 46XX karyotype, some 45XO karyotype).
- LHRH test (q.v.). This will establish if the hypothalamo-pituitary-gonadal axis is intact, and exclude primary gonadal failure.
- X-ray the left wrist for bone age. Look for delayed bone age in most causes of delayed puberty.

Q6: What treatment options are appropriate?

A6

- If the diagnosis is familial delayed puberty, the girl can be reassured that she will achieve a final adult height within the range predicted by her parents' heights.
- Girls with Turner syndrome need genetic counselling.
- If a systemic illness is diagnosed, then specific treatment will be required.
- Anorexia nervosa is a life-threatening condition that needs specialist child psychiatry input.

👫 OSCE counselling cases

OSCE COUNSELLING CASE 1.1 – Can you give my son something to make him taller?

This is a common question asked by parents of short and not-so-short children.

- Children who are 'short normal' – i.e. due to familial short stature or constitutional short stature – do not need treatment other than reassurance that they are healthy. Trials of growth hormone in short normal children have not shown any appreciable increase in final adult height. Growth hormone is indicated for growth hormone deficiency, Turner syndrome, Prader–Willi syndrome, Russell–Silver syndrome and in chronic renal failure.

- If growth hormone is indicated, the child and parents should be counselled about its use. Growth hormone is administered by daily subcutaneous injection until the child's height velocity falls below 2 cm per year (usually until mid-late teens).

- The family may wish to contact a parent support group such as the Child Growth Foundation.

- Regular monitoring of the child's growth is required to assess compliance and the effects of treatment.

- Many children with isolated growth hormone deficiency recover normal growth hormone secretion by puberty. They all need retesting at the end of the growth period.

- The benefit of exogenous growth hormone in growth hormone-deficient adults is controversial; there is some evidence that it improves general well-being and cardiac muscle contractility. However, this must be balanced against the cost of this very expensive drug.

OSCE COUNSELLING CASE 1.2 – Why is my child overweight?

Children are often brought to general paediatric clinics because of obesity.

- Find out in the history if there is any indication of pathology such as tiredness and lethargy in hypothyroidism, growth failure in Cushing's syndrome (very rare in children). Enquire about diet and exercise, and look at the phenotype of the parents (are the parents overweight as well?).

- Measure blood pressure, assess fat distribution (uniform in exogenous obesity), abdominal striae, acanthosis nigricans (sign of insulin resistance).

- The most likely diagnosis is exogenous obesity. This frequently induces more rapid growth and some advance in bone age. The family needs to be reassured that there is no underlying pathology.

- Explain that weight is determined by the balance of calorie intake and energy expenditure.

- Give dietary advice to reduce the fat content in the diet, reduce salt and increase fibre.

- Give exercise advice and suggest 30 minutes of exercise that makes the child breathless, every day.

- Set realistic targets for weight, and give positive encouragement.

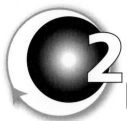

Developmental delay

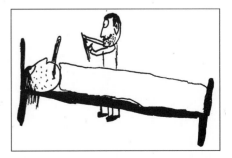

? Questions for each of the clinical cases

Q1: What is the likely differential diagnosis?
Q2: What issues in the given history support the diagnosis?
Q3: What additional features in the history would you seek to support a particular diagnosis?
Q4: What clinical examination would you perform and why?
Q5: What investigations would be most helpful and why?
Q6: What treatment options are appropriate?

Clinical cases

● CASE 2.1 – My newborn baby is very 'floppy' (hypotonic).

A 2-day-old baby is noted to have very poor tone and is floppy (like a rag doll). He is feeding rather slowly, but there are no other symptoms. The limbs move spontaneously.

● CASE 2.2 – My 9-month-old baby is not yet sitting and has stiff arms and legs.

A 9-month-old girl has been increasingly noted to hold her arms and legs out straight, with occasional crossing-over of the legs at the ankles. She does not sit unsupported, nor does she roll over effectively. She was born 12 weeks premature and was very ill during the neonatal period.

● CASE 2.3 – My 2-year-old daughter does not say any recognizable words.

A 2-year-old girl who is otherwise developing normally does not say any words which are recognizable. She is a third child, and her siblings' speech development was normal.

OSCE Counselling Cases

OSCE COUNSELLING CASE 2.1 – **My 16-month-old son is not yet walking.**

OSCE COUNSELLING CASE 2.2 – **My newborn baby has been diagnosed with Down's syndrome. What does this mean for her?**

🔑 Key concepts

In order to work through the core clinical cases in this chapter, you will need to understand the following key concepts.

Normal infant development

- From birth, babies develop new skills as they get older.
- These skills can be divided into five main groups: Gross motor (e.g. sitting, walking); (ii) Fine motor (e.g. holding an object, drawing a shape); (iii) Hearing and speech; (iv) Cognitive (thinking, understanding); and (v) Social (interaction with others).

Developmental milestones

- These are specific skills that *most* infants will achieve by a certain age (e.g. smiling to social overtures at 6 weeks of age, sitting unsupported at 8 months of age).
- Milestones are subdivided into the major development groups described above. It must be emphasized that although most infants will achieve milestones around the same time, some milestones will have a significant variation (e.g. walking unsupported usually occurs around 13 months, but may be achieved as early as 11 months or as late as 18 months in normal children).

Developmental delay

- This is defined as a significant delay in achieving developmental milestones which is outside the normal variation.
- Delay may occur in one, some or all of the developmental skills groups.

Cerebral palsy

- Cerebral palsy (CP) is a chronic disorder of muscle tone and movement due to a non-progressive injury to the developing brain.
- CP can result from a number of conditions that result in brain injury which particularly affects the motor areas of the brain.
- The events which lead to injury usually occur before, during or shortly after birth, but may be acquired at a later period following head trauma or meningitis. Most CP is due to brain injury which is acquired before birth.
- Infants may be floppy at birth and develop neonatal seizures. CP characteristically presents with motor delay and muscle stiffness (hypertonia or spasticity). If only the legs are affected, this is called diplegia; if the arm and leg on one side are affected, this is known as hemiplegia; and if all four limbs are affected the condition is known as quadriplegia.

Answers

CASE 2.1 – My newborn baby is very 'floppy' (hypotonic).

Q1: What is the likely differential diagnosis?

A1

- Non-paralytic conditions (e.g. chromosomal disorders [Down's syndrome], birth trauma or asphyxia, metabolic disorders, benign congenital hypotonia).

- Sepsis.

- Paralytic conditions (e.g. spinal muscular atrophy, congenital myopathy, myotonic dystrophy, myaesthenia gravis).

Q2: What issues in the given history support the diagnosis?

A2

This baby is moving the limbs spontaneously, and anti-gravity movements or maintenance of the posture of an elevated limb would strongly suggest that the baby is not paralysed. Therefore, a non-paralytic cause for the hypotonia is likely.

Q3: What additional features in the history would you seek to support a particular diagnosis?

A3

- Check pregnancy history – did the baby move normally in-utero, screening investigations (e.g. increased Down's risk).

- Check birth history – fetal distress, Apgar scores, need for resuscitation. Past obstetric history and family history – previous floppy babies or early neonatal deaths.

Q4: What clinical examination would you perform, and why?

A4

- Examine limb movements and check tendon reflexes to exclude a paralytic condition.

- Examine for dysmorphic features, e.g. those seen in Down's syndrome (see below) and cerebral irritability (e.g. jitteriness, seizures).

- Is the baby unwell? – unresponsive, mottled skin, tachypnoeic – which may suggest sepsis or a metabolic condition.

Q5: What investigations would be most helpful, and why?

A5

- Karyotype (if dysmorphism noted).

- Full blood count, electrolytes, blood culture, blood gas (? acidosis), urine culture, lumbar puncture (if baby is unwell).

- Cranial ultrasound (if birth trauma or asphyxia suspected).

- N.B. In paralytic conditions other investigations such as muscle biopsy, nerve conduction. studies and electromyography may be required to establish the diagnosis.

 Q6: What treatment options are appropriate?

A6

Treatment depends on the underlying cause of the hypotonia.

 CASE 2.2 – My 9-month-old baby is not yet sitting and has stiff arms and legs.

 Q1: What is the likely differential diagnosis?

A1

- Cerebral palsy.
- Metabolic disorder.
- Neuromuscular disorder.

Q2: What issues in the given history support the diagnosis?

A2

- The symptoms are suggestive of spastic quadriplegia.
- Preterm babies are much more likely to develop cerebral palsy than those born at term.

Q3: What additional features in the history would you seek to support a particular diagnosis?

A3

- Details of the neonatal course including condition at birth, need for ventilation, episodes of sepsis (particularly meningitis), abnormal cranial ultrasound scans, seizures. Family history (e.g. inherited disorder).

- Subsequent progress – poor head control at term, delayed developmental milestones (e.g. sucking, smiling). Hearing loss, visual problems (including abnormal eye movements – strabismus).

Q4: What clinical examination would you perform, and why?

A4

- Assess posture and muscle tone (? hypertonia/spasticity).

- Check tendon reflexes (? hyperreflexic).

- Look for hand preference when reaching out for objects and head lag. Infants should use both hands equally.

- Preservation of primitive reflexes (e.g. Moro). The Moro reflex is characterized by abduction and then adduction of the arms in response to gently allowing the head to fall a few centimetres (with appropriate support). It is normal in newborns but should not persist beyond 4 months of age. Other primitive reflexes include suck, grasp and asymmetric tonic neck reflexes.

 Q5: What investigations would be most helpful, and why?

A5

- The diagnosis of cerebral palsy is usually made on clinical grounds.

- MRI scanning may be of use (particularly if the neonatal cranial ultrasound was abnormal).

- If metabolic or myopathic disorders are suspected, then more specific investigations are warranted.

 Q6: What treatment options are appropriate?

A6

- Physiotherapy. This is the mainstay of treatment in order to prevent limb deformities and promote, as much as possible, maximal potential for motor development.

- Drug treatment (e.g. baclofen) for severe spasticity.

- Aids such as Piedro boots, walking frames or wheelchair may be necessary.

- Further multidisciplinary input, e.g. from speech therapists, dieticians, surgeons, pre-school teachers, educational psychologists, etc., may be required as the child gets older.

- Need for Statement of Special Educational Needs, and mainstream school inclusion.

● **CASE 2.3 – My 2-year-old daughter does not say any recognizable words.**

 Q1: What is the likely differential diagnosis?

A1

- Maturational language delay.

- Hearing impairment.

- Developmental language disorder.

- Mental retardation.

- Psychosocial deprivation.

- Autism.

 Q2: What issues in the given history support the diagnosis?

A2

The fact that she has otherwise normal development would make mental retardation and autism much less likely.

Q3: What additional features in the history would you seek to support a particular diagnosis?

A3

- Ask about pregnancy (? congenital infections), birth history (? birth asphyxia, sepsis) and early development including responses to sounds and voices.

- Ask about infant illnesses, especially meningitis and recurrent ear infections (e.g. otitis media) and exposure to ototoxic drugs (e.g. gentamicin).

- Did she pass the routine neonatal audiological screening? Is she socially responsive and does she attempt to copy sounds?

- Ask about family history of deafness and/or language delay. Enquire about potential psychosocial stresses within the family.

- Is there a failure of comprehension; e.g. can she follow a command?

- Is there a problem with the production of sounds?

- Can her parents understand her? Does she use non-verbal communication to demonstrate her needs?

 Q4: What clinical examination would you perform, and why?

A4

- Plot height, weight and head circumference on centile charts.

- Examine development milestones in other areas particularly social.

- Examine tympanic membranes for evidence of chronic otitis media (glue ear).

Q5: What investigations would be most helpful, and why?

A5

- Audiological assessment.

- Speech and language therapy assessment.

 Q6: What treatment options are appropriate?

A6

- Maturational delay is the most common cause of delayed speech, and the prognosis for this without specific treatment is excellent.

- If hearing impairment is detected, then treatment to improve hearing (e.g. grommets for otitis media or hearing aids for sensorineural deafness) should be instituted urgently in order to facilitate language development. Specific speech therapy may also be required.

👥 OSCE counselling cases

OSCE COUNSELLING CASE 2.1 – **My 16-month-old son is not yet walking.**

- Delayed walking is not uncommon.

- Children may employ alternative means of getting around (e.g. crawling, bottom shuffling). This may run in families.

- Occasionally, delayed walking may be related to problems such as muscular dystrophy or cerebral palsy (q.v.), but if other motor milestones (such as sitting, crawling and standing with support) have been reached and the legs are normal on examination (muscle bulk and tone, reflexes) these conditions are very unlikely.

- Most children will be walking by 18 months of age.

OSCE COUNSELLING CASE 2.2 – **My newborn baby has been diagnosed with Down's syndrome.**

What does this mean for her?

- Down's syndrome (DS, Trisomy 21) is the commonest chromosomal abnormality.

- Individuals with DS have an extra chromosome 21. This happened at some stage prior to fertilization. Although it is more common in older mothers, the precise cause is not known.

- Sometimes not all of the cells have an extra chromosome; this is called mosaicism.

- DS is not preventable, but there are tests that can be done during pregnancy; screening tests which may indicate an increased risk of the fetus having DS and diagnostic tests which confirm the condition (karyotype).

- Individuals with DS have certain physical characteristics which are usually recognizable at birth. These include: characteristic facies (upslanting eyes, wide palpebral fissure, prominent tongue); hypotonia; flattened occiput; single palmar creases, curved fifth finger, wide space between first and second toes (sandal gap); white spots on the iris (Brushfield spots).

- Associated with a degree of developmental delay (although most milestones are reached eventually).

- Mild to moderate learning difficulties (IQ variable, but usually > 80).

- Early feeding difficulties may be encountered.

- There is an increased incidence of congenital anomalies (particularly cardiac lesions and duodenal atresia).

- Some people with DS attend normal school initially and live fulfilling lives, including employment and relationships.

- Life expectancy is reduced (particularly if there are associated congenital anomalies), but people with DS can now live into their fifties.

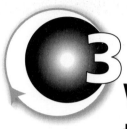

3

Weight faltering (failure to thrive)

Questions

Clinical cases

Key concepts

Answers

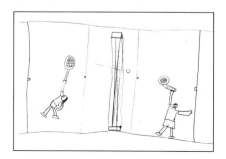

? Questions for each of the clinical cases

Q1: What is the likely differential diagnosis?
Q2: What issues in the given history support the diagnosis?
Q3: What additional features in the history would you seek to support a particular diagnosis?
Q4: What clinical examination would you perform, and why?
Q5: What investigations would be most helpful, and why?
Q6: What treatment options are appropriate?

Clinical cases

● CASE 3.1 – My 2-year-old son is not gaining weight.

A 2-year-old boy was on the 25th centile at birth; his weight is now on the 0.4th centile. On visiting the child's home, the health visitor notes that the members of the family eat separately, with no regular meal times. The child drinks 10–15 cups of orange squash per day. Food is put in front of him, but he refuses to eat after 2–3 mouthfuls.

● CASE 3.2 – My 18-month-old daughter is refusing to eat.

A mother is very concerned about her 18-month-old girl who is refusing to eat. The child clamps her mouth shut when offered food, and the mother often has to force-feed her, which makes her cough and splutter. Her weight has fallen from the 50th centile at birth to the 3rd centile. The girl's stools are loose, green and mucus-covered.

● CASE 3.3 – My 3-month-old is not gaining weight with breast feeding.

A 3-month-old breast-fed baby's weight was on the 25th centile at birth, but has dropped to the 10th centile now. The baby's length and head circumference are on the 10th centile.

👫 OSCE counselling cases

OSCE COUNSELLING CASE 3.1 – My 18-month-old son refuses to eat.

OSCE COUNSELLING CASE 3.2 – Should I bottle-feed my 3-month-old who is not gaining weight on breast milk?

Key concepts

In order to work through the core clinical cases in this chapter, you will need to understand the following key concepts.

Weight faltering (failure to thrive)

This is a descriptive term, not a diagnosis. No objective definition exists; the best available is "... a failure of expected growth". In clinical practice, classification usually rests on weight falling down two or more centiles. However:

- 5 per cent of normal children will shift down two or more centiles between birth and one year of age.

- 5 per cent of children on the 98th centile at birth shift down three centiles by six weeks.

- The commonest cause of weight faltering is under nutrition. Organic causes are identified in only 5 per cent of cases.

- 5 per cent of cases involve child protection issues.

Though rare, organic causes include:

- Inability to feed, e.g. cleft palate, oropharyngeal incoordination in neurodevelopmental delay.

- Inadequate retention of intake, e.g. vomiting, gastro-oesophageal reflux (q.v.).

- Malabsorption:

  - Fat, e.g. cystic fibrosis (q.v.)

  - Carbohydrate, e.g. coeliac disease (q.v.), lactose intolerance

  - Protein, e.g. cows' milk protein intolerance.

- Chronic illness, e.g. cardiac, respiratory, renal, liver or thyroid disease, malignancy.

Answers

 CASE 3.1 – My 2-year-old son is not gaining weight.

Q1: What is the likely differential diagnosis?

A1

- undernutrition due to poor feeding behaviour.
- poor feeding drive.
- gastro-oesophageal reflux.
- chronic illness
    - cystic fibrosis
    - renal disease
    - congenital heart disease
    - malignancy
    - hypothyroidism.
- malabsorption, e.g. cows' milk protein intolerance.

Social deprivation is not thought to be a factor in aetiology, although often stated in referrals.

Q2: What issues in the given history support the diagnosis?

A2

A large intake of squash with lack of regular family mealtimes suggests under-nutrition due to poor feeding behaviour.

Q3: What additional features in the history would you seek to support a particular diagnosis?

A3

A fall through two or more centiles, or weight <0.4th centile, should trigger an evaluation at home by a health visitor with observation of mealtimes with reference to:

- Content and frequency of meals recorded in a food diary.
- Interactions between different carers.
- The child's inherent feeding drive and appetite.
- Any evidence of difficulty swallowing or chewing (oromotor dysfunction).

- Medical staff need to take a detailed history, including a comprehensive systems review of any cardiorespiratory, gastrointestinal, urinary or neurodevelopmental symptoms with a detailed family and social history.

Q4: What clinical examination would you perform, and why?

A4

- Look at the growth pattern and assess neurodevelopment.
- Search for evidence of organic disease by performing a thorough physical examination.
- Search for:
  - Nutritional status.
  - Dysmorphism, e.g. congenital infection.
  - Clubbing, e.g. in cystic fibrosis.
  - Pallor.
  - Thyroid status.
  - Signs of congenital heart disease, e.g. cyanosis, murmur.
  - Chest deformity, added sounds (cystic fibrosis).
  - Abdominal masses (malignancy).

Q5: What investigations would be most helpful, and why?

A5

Investigations are only indicated if suggested by clinical assessment, and should be conducted early in management to minimize hospital attendance. Investigations that might be considered include:

- Full blood count and ferritin: for anaemia.
- Urea and electrolytes, creatinine: for renal disease.
- Thyroid function tests: for hypothyroidism.
- Coeliac antibodies: for coeliac disease.
- Urinalysis: for renal disease and urinary tract infections.

Q6: What treatment options are appropriate?

A6

The multidisciplinary team is the key to dietary and behavioural management. The doctor's role is to identify and advise about coincident medical conditions, and particularly to reassure if none is found. Dieticians and health visitors need to work with the family to:

- Establish regular family meal-times.

- Encourage intake of high-energy foods.
- Reduce fluid intake, especially of squash.
- Discourage force-feeding.

CASE 3.2 – My 18-month-old daughter is refusing to eat.

Q1: What is the likely differential diagnosis?

A1

- undernutrition due to poor feeding behaviour
- poor feeding drive
- gastro-oesophageal reflux
- chronic illness (as in Case 3.1)
- malabsorption, e.g. cows' milk protein intolerance.

Q2: What issues in the given history support the diagnosis?

A2

- Significant weight loss requires investigation. Force-feeding suggests poor feeding behaviour.
- Cough and spluttering when fed suggests oromotor dysfunction, gastro-oesophageal reflux, or a tracheo-oesophageal fistula.
- The consistency and colour of the stools suggests malabsorption or starvation stools.

Q3: What additional features in the history would you seek to support a particular diagnosis?

A3

- Content and frequency of meals recorded in a food diary.
- Interactions between different carers.
- The child's inherent feeding drive and appetite.
- Any evidence of difficult swallowing or chewing (oromotor dysfunction).
- Respiratory symptoms.
- Vomiting.
- Medical staff need to take a detailed history, including a comprehensive systems review of any cardiorespiratory, gastrointestinal, urinary or neurodevelopmental symptoms with a detailed family and social history.

Q4: What clinical examination would you perform, and why?

A4

● Look at the growth pattern and assess neurodevelopment.

● Search for evidence of organic disease by performing a thorough physical examination (see above).

 Q5: What investigations would be most helpful, and why?

A5

● Once again, investigations are only indicated if suggested by clinical assessment, and should be conducted early in management to minimize hospital attendance and over-reliance on an organic solution to the problem. Investigations that might be considered in addition to those listed above include:

  ● Stool analysis: for microscopy and culture, virology and faecal-1-elastase (a measure of fat malabsorption).

  ● Sweat test (q.v.): to exclude cystic fibrosis in very young children or where a history of malabsorption or respiratory symptoms exists.

  ● Chromosome analysis: in girls, for Turner syndrome (q.v.).

  ● Barium swallow or pH study: to rule out tracheo-oesophageal fistula and gastro-oesophageal reflux (q.v.).

 Q6: What treatment options are appropriate?

A6

● A community-based multidisciplinary team is the key to dietary and behavioural management.

● In addition to a dietician and health visitor, this family may need a child psychologist to advise on a feeding behaviour modification programme, and a speech therapist to assess and advise on swallowing, oromotor skills, feeding technique and introduction of foods of different textures.

● CASE 3.3 – My 3-month-old is not gaining weight with breast feeding.

Q1: What is the likely differential diagnosis?

A1

● Normal growth pattern – 'catch-down' growth.

● Undernutrition – inadequate intake with breast feeding.

● Oromotor dysfunction – usually has an underlying cause, e.g. developmental delay, cleft lip and palate.

● Organic disease (see list in Key Concepts).

Q2: What issues in the given history support the diagnosis?

A2

● The history, and symmetrical growth suggests catch-down growth.

● Breast feeding and oromotor function needs further assessment.

 Q3: What additional features in the history would you seek to support a particular diagnosis?

A3

Seek further information about:

● Pregnancy, birth history.

● Mother's health and nutritional status.

● Intercurrent symptoms – vomiting, diarrhoea, chest symptoms.

● Feeding patterns and swallowing.

● Neurodevelopmental milestones.

Q4: What clinical examination would you perform, and why?

A4

Search for:

● Growth pattern.

● Nutritional status.

● Dysmorphism.

● Pallor.

● Thyroid status.

● Signs of congenital heart disease.

● Chest deformity, added sounds.

● Abdominal masses.

● Neurodevelopmental assessment.

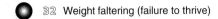

Q5: What investigations would be most helpful, and why?

A5

- Investigations are only indicated if suggested by clinical assessment.
- If catch-down growth is diagnosed clinically, urinalysis is the only investigation necessary.

Q6: What treatment options are appropriate?

A6

Families often require much reassurance that the growth pattern is normal, and follow-up – ideally in a community-based setting with the health visitor – is advised.

ᵔᵔ OSCE counselling cases

OSCE COUNSELLING CASE 3.1 – My 18-month-old son refuses to eat.

An 18-month-old boy has a long history of refusing to eat. He takes one or two mouthfuls and then refuses, and starts to have a tantrum. His weight has fallen from the 10th to below the 0.4th centile. His parents say that they are at the end of their tether. A full history, physical examination and investigations do not reveal an organic cause.

Weight faltering is usually a problem of feeding behaviour, and not due to serious illnesses which have been excluded by a thorough examination and tests. The problem is not the parents' or the child's fault, and is very common. Force-feeding makes the problem worse. Several members of the health team are needed to help:

- The dietician will assess what the boy does eat, and will advise on a variety of high-calorie foods.

- The health visitor will visit the family at home and advise on establishing regular meal times, and on the need for all family members to have a consistent approach to feeding the child.

- A child psychologist may be useful to assess child development and advise on a behaviour programme and on communication with children.

- A speech therapist may be useful to assess swallowing, oromotor skills, feeding technique and introduction of foods of different textures.

OSCE COUNSELLING CASE 3.2 – Should I bottle-feed my 3-month-old who is not gaining weight on breast milk?

A breast-fed, 3-month-old baby's weight has fallen from the 25th centile at birth to the 10th centile. He is otherwise healthy and his head circumference and length are on the 10th centile. Clinical assessment does not reveal an organic cause, and 'catch-down' growth is diagnosed.

- Your baby is healthy.

- Thorough assessment has ruled out a serious disease.

- Tests would only be needed if we had concerns after checking your baby.

- The baby's growth pattern is called 'catch-down' growth.

- Birth weight reflects placental function.

- Weight in babies reflects nutritional intake, and if this if good – as it is in your case – it also reflects genetic potential.

- The baby's growth needs to be monitored by the health visitor.

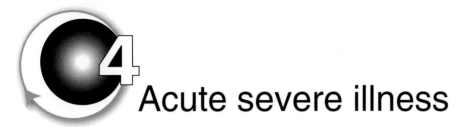

Acute severe illness

Questions

Clinical cases

Key concepts

Answers

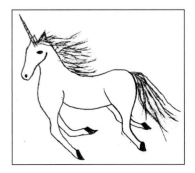

? Questions for each of the clinical cases

Q1: What is the likely differential diagnosis?
Q2: What issues in the given history support the diagnosis?
Q3: What additional features in the history would you seek to support a particular diagnosis?
Q4: What clinical examination would you perform, and why?
Q5: What investigations would be most helpful, and why?
Q6: What treatment options are appropriate?

Clinical cases

● CASE 4.1 – My 6-month-old baby has a cough, is burning up, and is struggling to breathe.

A 6-month-old baby has had a cold for the past few days, but in the past 12 hours has developed a high fever, cough, poor feeding and loose stools. He has vomited twice and is restlessly sleeping more than usual or is crying inconsolably.

● CASE 4.2 – My 2-day-old baby is blue and can't breathe.

A 2-day-old baby looks dusky and is having difficulty breathing. He has not been feeding well, and has been sweaty. A murmur was heard at birth.

● CASE 4.3 – My 5-month-old isn't breathing.

A 5-month-old baby is found in its cot, not breathing, 1 hour after being put down to sleep.

⚇ OSCE counselling cases

OSCE COUNSELLING CASE 4.1 – **My child is hot; has she got meningitis?**

OSCE COUNSELLING CASE 4.2 – **My toddler has diarrhoea and vomiting; what should I do?**

Key concepts

In order to work through the core clinical cases in this chapter, you will need to understand the following key concepts.

Children are not small adults

Key differences are:

- Size: This changes rapidly in the first year of life. An average birth weight of 3 kg increases to 10 kg by 1 year. Between the ages of 1 year and 10 years, weight can be predicted by the formula: Weight (kg) = 2 × (age [years] + 4).

- Anatomy: younger children have a short, soft neck: the upper airway tends to obstruct if the neck is overextended in resuscitation.

- Physiology: Normal physiological parameters (pulse, respiratory rate, blood pressure) change with age.

  - Infants aged under 6 months are obligate nasal breathers; upper respiratory infections can cause respiratory embarrassment and feeding difficulties.

  - Small airways: resistance to flow is inversely proportional to the fourth power of the airway radius, so minimal airway inflammation and swelling can cause significant obstruction.

- Psychology: Children fear illnesses and emergencies through a lack of prior knowledge, a magical concept of illness (they may think illness has been caused by something they thought or did), picking up on parental anxiety, and professional failure to communicate at the child's level.

Parents find acute illnesses in children terrifying. Parents of young children, through an understandable fear of meningitis and septicaemia, often seek medical reassurance for symptoms (e.g. fever, cough) that professionals consider being minor and self-limiting.

Algorithms exist for recognition of the sick child, basic and advanced paediatric life support and choking.

Investigations in acute severe illness

Specific investigations are guided by the history and examination, but often these are vague and/or non-specific. In these circumstances it is appropriate to perform the following in an acutely unwell child.

- Full blood count: risk of serious bacterial infection is increased if white cell count (WCC) is $>15 \times 10^9$/litre or is reduced (especially in newborns), or there is an abnormal platelet count.

- Urea and electrolytes – for electrolyte disturbance.

- C-reactive protein (CRP) – is an acute-phase protein, the levels of which may rise in serious bacterial infection.

- Blood cultures.

- Blood sugar – hypoglycaemia may suggest poor intake or inborn error of metabolism.

- Urinalysis – positive nitrite test and/or Leucostix is suggestive of urinary tract infection and needs confirmation by urgent microscopy and subsequent culture.

- Lumbar puncture (LP): cerebrospinal fluid (CSF) microscopy confirms or excludes meningitis in 80 per cent of cases. Lumbar puncture should be deferred if there are *signs* of cerebral herniation (raised intracranial pressure *cannot* be excluded by CT scan), focal neurological signs, or cardiorespiratory compromise, but empirical antibiotic therapy should be given without delay. A delayed LP can confirm the diagnosis of meningitis, as the cellular and biochemical changes remain in CSF up to 44–68 hours after the start of antibiotic treatment. CSF microscopy and PCR for *Meningococcus* and *Pneumococcus* from delayed LP can guide subsequent treatment, although cultures may be negative within 2–6 h of antibiotic administration.

Answers

 CASE 4.1 – **My 6-month-old baby has a cough, is burning up and is struggling to breathe.**

 Q1: What is the likely differential diagnosis?

A1

- Septicaemia.
- Meningitis.
- Lower respiratory tract infection.
- Gastroenteritis and shock.
- Urinary tract infection.
- Hypoglycaemia.
- Inborn error of metabolism.

Q2: What issues in the given history support the diagnosis?

A2

- An acute illness in young children often presents with non-specific symptoms. Septicaemia must be considered in all infants presenting with fever, drowsiness and poor feeding. The baby's clinical condition has deteriorated rapidly during the previous 12 hours.
- Meningitis is suggested by irritability and inconsolable crying.
- Vomiting and diarrhoea suggest gastroenteritis.
- Urinary tract infection can present with non-specific symptoms like this.
- Inborn errors of metabolism are rare, but should be considered.

Q3: What additional features in the history would you seek to support a particular diagnosis?

A3

- Rapid clinical assessment of airway, breathing, circulation and disability (see below) may indicate the need to intervene urgently before taking a detailed history.
- Septicaemia, meningitis and urinary tract infection are difficult to diagnose on history in infants, and should be considered in all young children with acute severe illness.

- Diarrhoea and vomiting needs assessment of the duration and frequency of symptoms, fluid intake, urine output and presence of bile or blood in vomit or stool.

- A history of consanguinity or previous sudden death in childhood may suggest an inborn error of metabolism.

Q4: What clinical examination would you perform, and why?

A4

- Perform a rapid clinical assessment of airway, breathing (work of breathing, respiratory rate, stridor, wheeze, cyanosis), circulation (tachycardia, weak pulse volume, prolonged capillary refill time, pallor or cool peripheries, petechial rash) and conscious level. In the absence of cardiorespiratory compromise or deterioration and a normal conscious level, a more detailed secondary examination is undertaken seeking:

  - General inspection: fever, rashes.

  - Cardiovascular: heart murmurs, signs of heart failure (tachycardia, gallop rhythm, palpable liver).

  - Respiratory: wheeze, stridor, air entry on auscultation.

  - Abdomen: hepatosplenomegaly (suggesting an inborn error of metabolism), abdominal swelling or masses, increased or 'tinkling' bowel sounds (suggesting intestinal obstruction, e.g. intussusception q.v.).

  - Neurology: the 'classic signs' of meningitis are absent under 1 year of age. Irritability and a bulging fontanelle may suggest meningitis, but their absence does not exclude it.

Q5: What investigations would be most helpful, and why?

A5

- Full blood count.

- Urea and electrolytes.

- C-reactive protein (CRP).

- Blood cultures.

- Blood sugar.

- Urinalysis.

- Lumbar puncture (LP).

Q6: What treatment options are appropriate?

A6

- Maintain airway.

- Oxygen in as high a concentration as can be delivered (in hospital, usually 15 L/min via a mask with a rebreathe bag).

- Intravenous access for i.v. antibiotics and fluids.

- Rapid bolus of 0.9 per cent saline to correct shock.

- Maintenance fluids plus deficit to correct dehydration infused over the next 24–48 hours.

- Admit to hospital for observation, supportive treatment and intravenous antibiotics, and observation until culture results known.

CASE 4.2 – My 2-day-old baby is blue and can't breathe.

Q1: What is the likely differential diagnosis?

A1

- Congenital heart disease, e.g. transposition of the great arteries.

- Lower respiratory tract infection.

- Neonatal septicaemia.

- Urinary tract infection.

- Inborn error of metabolism.

Q2: What issues in the given history support the diagnosis?

A2

- Murmur at birth, sweatiness, poor feeding, and cyanosis suggest congenital heart disease. The ductus arteriosus closes within hours or a few days of age, suggesting a duct-dependent lesion (q.v.).

- Lower respiratory tract infection is suggested by the history of difficulty breathing.

- Neonatal sepsis is suggested by the age of the baby. Meningitis, septicaemia, urinary tract infection and inborn error of metabolism may present with non-specific symptoms in newborns and young children.

Q3: What additional features in the history would you seek to support a particular diagnosis?

A3

- Seek antenatal history, including details of antenatal scans and family history of congenital heart disease.

- Neonatal sepsis is suggested by history of maternal fever, prolonged rupture of membranes, prematurity, maternal carriage of group B streptococci.

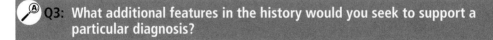

- Birth history and a history of feeding from birth is important.

Q4: What clinical examination would you perform, and why?

A4

- Rapid clinical assessment of airway, breathing, circulation and disability (see below) may indicate the need to intervene urgently before taking a detailed history.
- Seek clinical signs of congenital heart disease (cyanosis, tachycardia, gallop rhythm, heart murmur, absent femoral pulses or bounding pulse volume, hepatomegaly, tachypnoea).
- Measure oxygen saturation in air and in 100 per cent oxygen, using pulse oximetry.

 Q5: What investigations would be most helpful, and why?

A5

In addition to investigations for sepsis (see Case 1.1, A5), consider:

- ECG – for signs of congenital heart disease.
- Chest X-ray – for cardiomegaly, oligaemic or plethoric lung fields, signs of lower respiratory tract infection.
- Blood gas – in oxygen.
- Echocardiogram – for congenital heart disease.

Q6: What treatment options are appropriate?

A6

- Maintain airway.
- Oxygen.
- Intravenous access.
- Consider intravenous prostaglandin E_2 to maintain patency of ductus arteriosus.
- Intravenous antibiotics.
- Intravenous fluids and stop feeds pending definitive diagnosis and management.
- Consider transfer to regional paediatric cardiac unit (see also Chapter 7).

CASE 4.3 – My 5-month-old isn't breathing.

 Q1: What is the likely differential diagnosis?

A1

- Sudden Infant Death Syndrome (SIDS).

- Serious bacterial infection.

- Electrolyte disturbance, e.g. due to dehydration.

- Gastro-oesophageal reflux (q.v.).

- Seizures (q.v.).

- Upper airway obstruction.

- Cardiac anomaly or arrhythmia.

- Iatrogenic poisoning.

- Non-accidental injury.

 Q2: What issues in the given history support the diagnosis?

A2

Sudden Infant Death Syndrome (SIDS) is a diagnosis of exclusion; other causes may present in the same way and must be considered.

 Q3: What additional features in the history would you seek to support a particular diagnosis?

A3

Rapid clinical assessment of airway, breathing, circulation and disability (see below) may indicate the need to intervene urgently before taking a detailed history. Paediatric resuscitation is usually conducted by teams; one team member can be delegated to take a detailed history.

- Review of intercurrent symptoms and prior illness;

- Risk factors for SIDS should be reviewed and recorded, although identification of a single aetiology is impossible in most cases:

  - Modifiable factors:

    - Co-sleeping.

    - Bedding and clothing (evidence suggests increased risk from overheating but studies did not investigate the relationship between bedding, ambient temperature and amount of infant clothing).

    - Pre- and post-natal smoking.

  - Non-modifiable risk factors:

    - Young mother.

    - Low birth weight.

    - Prematurity.

    - No antenatal care.

- – Single mother.
- – High parity.
- – Low socio-economic class.
- – Admission to special care baby unit in infancy.
- Past history should include a check of any previous injuries and antenatal/birth history.
- Drug history should include a review of drugs which are kept in the home.
- Family history should include consanguinity, family history of infant deaths.
- Detailed social history, including review of housing and call to social services to check whether the child is on a child protection register.

Q4: What clinical examination would you perform, and why?

A4

- Rapid clinical assessment may indicate the need for immediate basic life support and advanced life support.

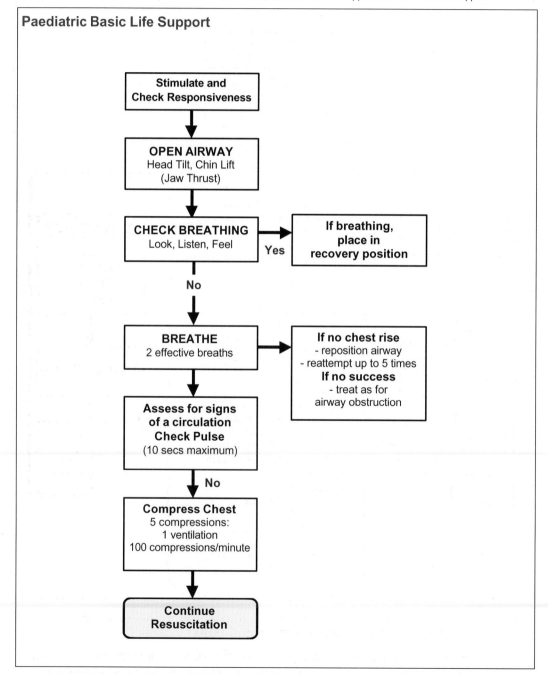

Paediatric Basic Life Support

```
          Stimulate and
      Check Responsiveness
                │
                ▼
          OPEN AIRWAY
        Head Tilt, Chin Lift
          (Jaw Thrust)
                │
                ▼
        CHECK BREATHING  ──────►   If breathing,
        Look, Listen, Feel            place in
                       Yes        recovery position
                │
               No
                │
                ▼
            BREATHE       ──────►   If no chest rise
        2 effective breaths        - reposition airway
                │                - reattempt up to 5 times
                │                    If no success
                │                     - treat as for
                ▼                   airway obstruction
        Assess for signs
        of a circulation
          Check Pulse
        (10 secs maximum)
                │
               No
                │
                ▼
         Compress Chest
        5 compressions:
          1 ventilation
      100 compressions/minute
                │
                ▼
            Continue
          Resuscitation
```

Reproduced with kind permission of The Resuscitation Council UK.

Paediatric Advanced Life Support

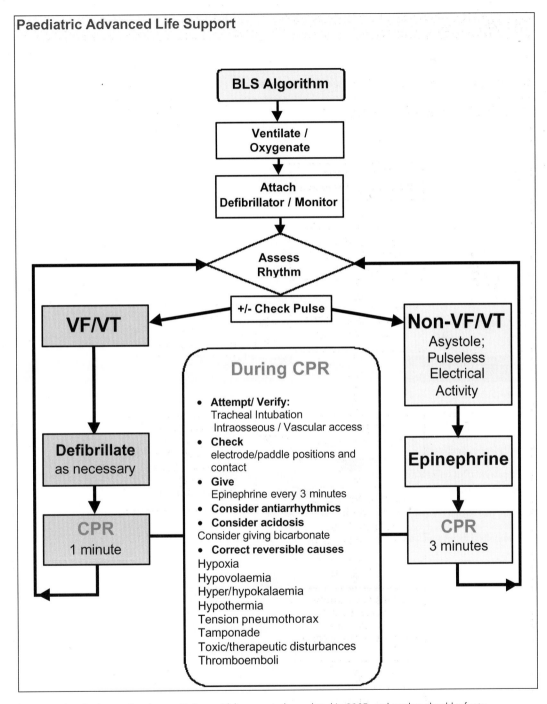

Important note: International resuscitation guidelines are to be updated in 2005, and readers should refer to www.resus.org.uk. Reproduced with kind permission of The Resuscitation Council UK.

- Physical examination following successful or during active resuscitation should include a search for cataracts (may occur in inborn errors of metabolism), congenital abnormalities, hepatosplenomegaly, presence of blood in nose or mouth, and signs of injury.

Q5: What investigations would be most helpful, and why?

A5

In addition to investigations for sepsis (see Case 1.1, A5), consider:

- Urinalysis (q.v.) – collect urine for screening for inborn error of metabolism and toxicology.

- Chest X-ray – for cardiomegaly, oligaemic or plethoric lung fields, signs of lower respiratory tract infection.

- Blood gas and pulse oximetry – in high-flow oxygen.

- Blood lactate, ammonia – for signs of inborn errors of metabolism.

- Nasopharyngeal aspirate, throat swab – for evidence of viral or bacterial infection.

- Skeletal survey – for unexplained injuries.

- Skin biopsy and blood – for inborn errors of metabolism.

- Electroencephalogram (EEG) – for seizures.

- Barium swallow or pH study – for gastro-oesophageal reflux.

- Cranial imaging – for intracranial trauma, bleeding, neoplasia, sepsis.

Q6: What treatment options are appropriate?

A6

- Basic and advanced paediatric life support.

- Intravenous antibiotics.

- Resuscitation is unlikely to be successful and is usually stopped if spontaneous circulation is not restored within 30 minutes of cumulative life support, except in cases of poisoning or hypothermia.

Following the sudden unexpected death of an infant, families need:

- counselling with verbal and written information about why their baby died;

- to be encouraged to see and hold the baby;

- to be informed that a coroner's post-mortem investigation is required by law in all such cases, and appropriate consent is taken;

- to be informed that the general practitioner, health visitor, police and social services will be involved; and

- offered bereavement support from other agencies and a follow-up visit at home.

ÅÅ OSCE counselling cases

OSCE COUNSELLING CASE 4.1 – My child is hot; has she got meningitis?

A 14-month-old girl presents with a 1-day history of fever, coryza and cough. A physical examination suggests an upper respiratory tract infection.

- Fear of meningitis is the commonest reason that parents of young children seek medical reassurance for self-limiting illnesses. Doctors and parents approach such illnesses from different perspectives. Doctors focus on diagnosis, whereas parents want to protect their children and alleviate symptoms. Parents are often made to feel that their demands are inappropriate.

- The doctor's attitude is important if we are to reassure parents; a thorough history and examination is essential. Parents are rightly suspicious if reassurance is given when the child hasn't been seen and examined.

Counselling should involve:

- The opportunity for the parents and the child to express their specific concerns.

- An explanation of each concern.

- Specific reassurance that serious illness has been ruled out.

- A specific diagnosis, if one has been made.

- Advice about which symptoms and signs to be concerned about, and when and where to seek medical help again.

OSCE COUNSELLING CASE 4.2 – My toddler has diarrhoea and vomiting; what should I do?

A 14-month-old boy has had diarrhoea and vomiting for 1 day. He has vomited twice today, and has had about six loose bowel motions. Rotavirus has been identified in the stool. The baby is systemically stable, without clinical evidence of shock or dehydration.

- The commonest causes of diarrhoea and vomiting in infants and small children is gastroenteritis (also known as 'tummy bug'). Most children with gastroenteritis will get better with no special treatment, although it can continue for up to 2 weeks.

- However, it is always taken seriously because babies and small children lose body fluid quickly and can become dehydrated. It is important to prevent this by giving lots of clear drinks (juice or Dioralyte) to replace the loss from the diarrhoea and vomiting. Give small sips frequently. (Dioralyte is a clear drink which contains minerals and sugar to replace those lost because of diarrhoea and vomiting. It is not a medicine and does not stop diarrhoea and vomiting.)

- Normal feeds should be started again after 24 hours.

- You must watch out for the signs of dehydration and go to the doctor if you see:

  - sunken eyes and a glazed look

  - mottled skin

  - strong-smelling urine

  - dry mouth

- Handwashing, after nappy changes and before making feeds or meals, is very important if you are to stop other family members from catching the virus.

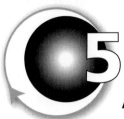

5 Acute and chronic fever

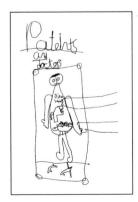

? Questions for each of the clinical cases

Q1: What is the likely differential diagnosis?
Q2: What issues in the given history support the given diagnosis?
Q3: What additional features in the given history would you seek to support a particular diagnosis?
Q4: What clinical examination would you perform, and why?
Q5: What investigations would be most helpful, and why?
Q6: What treatment options are appropriate?

Clinical cases

● CASE 5.1 – My 18-month-old has developed a fever and a rash.

She has recently become quieter than usual. After 2 days of fever she broke out in a rash.

● CASE 5.2 – My 4-year-old has developed a fever 2 weeks after returning to the UK from abroad.

We have just returned from Africa, where we had been working when he was born. He had uncomplicated chicken pox at 10 months, but has been otherwise well and is up to date with his immunizations.

● CASE 5.3 – My 3-year-old son has had a fever for 10 days, and his fingers are peeling.

He was seen by his GP with a 4-day history of intermittent high fever above 39°C, red eyes, sore throat and cervical lymphadenopathy. He initially had a rash that has now faded.

ⅲⅲ OSCE counselling cases

OSCE COUNSELLING CASE 5.1 – **My child has a rash and I am pregnant. What if it is German measles?**

OSCE COUNSELLING CASE 5.2 – **All my friends are advising me not to let my child have the MMR vaccine.**

Key concepts

In order to work through the core clinical cases in this chapter, you will need to understand the following key concepts.

Childhood infectious diseases

Infections are the most common cause of acute illness in children, and are responsible for about 14 million deaths in children worldwide each year.

- Morbidity and mortality from infections has fallen dramatically in developed countries as a consequence of improved living conditions, sanitation, immunization, antibiotic therapy and modern medical care.

- Some infections are still a major problem in some parts of the developed world, including meningococcal disease and tuberculosis.

- At birth, infants have a functioning immune system, but their circulating immunoglobulins, derived from their mother, decrease during the first few months of life, leaving them susceptible to common infections. These include the childhood exanthems (illnesses with fever and rash) measles, mumps, rubella, varicella (chicken pox), and roseola infantum (see also Chapter 12).

Rubella (German measles)

Rubella is usually a mild, self-limiting childhood illness.

- The incubation period is 14–21 days, and infection spread is usually by the respiratory route. There is a mild prodrome with a low-grade fever, followed by a maculopapular rash, starting on the face, then spreading to the whole body, and fading in 3–5 days. There may also be cervical lymphadenopathy, mild pharyngitis and conjunctivitis.

- Complications may include arthritis, encephalitis, thrombocytopaenia and myocarditis.

- The major complication is infection during pregnancy, when it can give rise to the Rubella syndrome in the developing fetus. This is the triad of congenital deafness, cardiac defects and cataracts, but it usually also includes severe mental retardation.

- Maternal infection during the first trimester is the most serious, when organogenesis is occurring, but the effects on the developing fetus progressively become less severe if infection occurs during the second or third trimesters.

Measles

Measles is a severe childhood illness with appreciable mortality, particularly in infants (see below).

- The incubation period is 10–12 days, and infection spread is by the respiratory route. The prodromal illness includes symptoms similar to the common cold, leading to a severe dry cough, fever, rhinorrhoea, conjunctivitis, and a macular rash starting behind the ears and progressing to the whole body. The rash lasts for 5–7 days and turns brown as it fades.

- Complications may include pneumonia, and rarely, subacute sclerosing panencephalitis (SSPE), a late complication which can result in neurodegeneration and death.

- Measles is making a resurgence in the UK in areas where the vaccination uptake has fallen below that required for 'herd immunity'.

KFCORLE

ECG
Aspirin
Ig

Anyeurysm
Thrombus
Ischaemia

Key concepts 55 ●

Kawasaki disease

This condition affects children, mainly from the age of 6 months to 4 years.

- Kawasaki disease is a vasculitic disease, affecting small and medium-sized vessels, including the coronary arteries in about one-third of children, which can lead to aneurysms. Subsequent narrowing of these vessels from scar formation can result in myocardial ischaemia and sudden death.

- The diagnosis is made clinically, requiring the presence of a fever and four out of five other criteria, or the presence of fever, three other criteria and coronary artery aneurysms on echocardiography.

- The fever must be persistent and spiking, for more than 5 days.

- The other criteria are: bilateral non-exudative conjunctivitis; oropharyngeal mucositis; a polymorphous rash; cervical lymphadenopathy; and changes in the extremities. These changes involve erythema and oedema on the wrists and ankles, desquamation of the skin round the nails, and peeling of the skin, which may include the perineum.

- Thrombocytosis is a late feature of the disease.

- Kawasaki disease is now known to be the result of a bacterial toxin acting as a superantigen.

- Treatment is by intravenous human immunoglobulin and aspirin to reduce the risk of coronary artery aneurysm and thrombus formation.

- Echocardiography is now required for all cases of suspected Kawasaki disease.

UK immunization schedule

Active immunization (vaccination) is the administration of inactivated or attenuated live organisms or their products to induce an immune response. Protection lasts for months or years, but takes weeks to develop and may be dependent on receiving more than one dose. The UK schedule is as follows:

- BCG and Hepatitis B in neonatal period to high-risk infants. Hepatitis B repeated at 1, 2 and 12 months.

- Diphtheria, tetanus, acellular pertussis, inactivated polio vaccine, *Haemophilus influenzae* (DTP/IPV/Hib) and *Meningococcus* C: three doses at 2, 3 and 4 months of age.

- Measles, Mumps and Rubella (MMR) at 12–15 months of age.

- DTP/IPV/Hib and MMR at 3–5 years.

- BCG at 10–14 years.

- Booster Diphtheria, Tetanus and Polio at 13–18 years.

Answers

● CASE 5.1 – **My 18-month-old has developed a mild fever and a rash.**

 Q1: What is the likely differential diagnosis?

A1

- Rubella.
- Measles.
- Roseola infantum.
- Kawasaki disease.
- Other causes of childhood infection, e.g. streptococcal and meningococcal infection.

 Q2: What issues in the given history support the diagnosis?

A2

The child is mildly unwell, which would suggest rubella. Measles causes a particularly unpleasant illness, with miserable, unwell children. A high fever and a toxic, unwell-looking child may occur with meningococcal disease or streptococcal infection.

 Q3: What additional features in the history would you seek to support a particular diagnosis?

A3

- Does the child have a sore throat (pharyngitis), or red eyes (conjunctivitis)?
- Is there any evidence of arthralgia, swollen glands in the neck, or history of a rash starting on the face?

Q4: What clinical examination would you perform, and why?

A4

- Check the temperature, heart rate and respiratory rate.
- Look at the rash – is it blanching, is it maculopapular?
- Look at the throat, eyes and tympanic membranes.
- Feel for the cervical and occipital lymph nodes.
- Assess the joints for pain and swelling.

Q5: What investigations would be most helpful, and why?

A5

Usually, rubella infection is a clinical diagnosis, and no investigations are necessary. If there were a risk for a pregnant contact, then rubella serology would be appropriate.

 Q6: What treatment options are appropriate?

A6

Symptomatic measures only are appropriate, e.g. paracetamol for fever. The rash in children is not usually itchy, unlike in adults.

CASE 5.2 – My 4-year-old has developed a fever 2 weeks after returning to the UK from Africa.

 Q1: What is the likely differential diagnosis?

A1

- Viral upper respiratory tract infection.
- Childhood exanthems such as rubella.
- Meningococcal disease.
- Consider malaria.

 Q2: What issues in the given history support the diagnosis?

A2

Any history of recent travel abroad must raise the possibility of malaria. For a child from Africa, this is likely to be severe *Falciparum* infection, presenting acutely with high fever. Children from South Asia tend to contract the milder *Vivax* form, which may present with intermittent fever. Ask about any evidence of severe infection, such as anorexia, not drinking, drowsiness, fits or rigors, or meningococcal rash. Malaria may present with intermittent rigors as the sporozoites enter the bloodstream.

Q3: What additional features in the history would you seek to support a particular diagnosis?

A3

Ask about a history of rigors. Find out whether the child and family took anti-malarial prophylaxis before, during and after their visit, and whether their drugs covered the sensitivities of the malaria parasites prevalent in their area. Look up the travel advice in the *British National Formulary*.

Q4: What clinical examination would you perform, and why?

A4

Look for a focus of infection, e.g.:

- Respiratory/ENT: coryza, cough, noisy or fast breathing.

- Gastrointestinal: vomiting, diarrhoea, abdominal pain.

- CNS: lethargy, irritability, photophobia.

- Genito-urinary: dysuria, smelly urine.

- Skin: rash, conjunctivitis, skin lesions.

- Musculoskeletal: joint pain.

Q5: What investigations would be most helpful, and why?

A5

- Measure temperature.

- Full blood count.

- Thick blood films at the point of rigor to identify malarial parasites.

- Blood culture.

 Q6: What treatment options are appropriate?

A6

- Paracetamol to reduce fever. Also use physical measures to cool the patient down, e.g. strip down to vest and pants, or use fan to circulate air in room but not directly on the child.

- If malaria is confirmed, include an antimalarial drug such as chloroquine. Check with your local microbiology service for guidance on the correct treatment depending on the sensitivities of the malarial parasite strain.

CASE 5.3 – My 3-year-old son has had a fever for 10 days, and his fingers are peeling.

Q1: What is the likely differential diagnosis?

A1

- Differential diagnosis of fever/rashes/sore throat.
- Kawasaki disease.
- Scarlet fever.
- Glandular fever.
- Group A streptococcal infection.
- Measles.
- Rubella.
- Roseola.
- Viral or bacterial tonsillitis.

Q2: What issues in the given history support the diagnosis?

A2

A history of prolonged fever persisting for more than 10 days, the changes in the oral cavity, rash on the skin, cervical lymphadenopathy, peeling of the skin on fingers and toes are strongly suggestive of Kawasaki disease.

Q3: What additional features in the history would you seek to support a particular diagnosis?

A3

- Ask how high the temperature has been; has it been continuous or spiking up and down?
- What sort of rash, and where did it start?
- Is there anyone else in the family affected (usually not with Kawasaki disease)?
- Has the child been fully vaccinated (should make measles and rubella less likely)?

Q4: What clinical examination would you perform, and why?

A4

- Examine the whole of the body for a rash.
- Look for Koplik's spots on the fauces (look like grains of salt on a red background seen in the early stages of measles).
- Strawberry tongue (scarlet fever).
- Palatal petechiae (may be seen in viral infections and meningococcal disease).
- Swelling or erythema of extremities (Kawasaki).
- Splenomegaly (glandular fever).

 Q5: What investigations would be most helpful, and why?

A5

- Full blood count: atypical lymphocytes in glandular fever. Increased platelets in Kawasaki.
- Monospot/Paul Bunnell test (for glandular fever).

  Kawasaki disease is mainly a clinical diagnosis, but the following can be suggestive:

- Raised platelet count ($< 500\,000/\text{mm}^3$). Blood culture.
- Erythrocyte sedimentation rate (ESR) very high.
- Echocardiogram for coronary artery aneurysms.
- Coronary artery aneurysms on echocardiography.

Q6: What treatment options are appropriate?

A6

- Treatment of Kawasaki disease is intravenous human immunoglobulin and aspirin to reduce risk of coronary artery aneurysm and thrombus formation.
- Follow-up by a paediatric cardiologist is essential, with repeat echocardiography performed about 6 weeks after the original episode.

👥 OSCE counselling cases

OSCE COUNSELLING CASE 5.1 – My child has a rash and I am pregnant. What if it is German measles?

- Rubella is a common childhood exanthem which is now very rare in the UK due to uptake of the MMR vaccine. The child is likely to have a rash from some other infection if he has been immunized.

- The mother is likely to have been vaccinated against rubella. All pregnant women have their rubella status checked at the booking visit, so it should be possible to find out her status.

- Check the child's vaccination status; if not known, take blood from mother and child for rubella serology.

- If the child has rubella infection and the mother is non-immune, action depends on the stage of pregnancy: the highest risk to the fetus is in the first trimester. The mother and father will require specialist counselling and consideration of the option of termination of pregnancy.

OSCE COUNSELLING CASE 5.2 – All my friends are advising me not to give my child MMR vaccine.

- Measles infection is a childhood killer and cause of considerable mortality (1 in 1000 under 1 year of age). It is also responsible for a rare fatal, degenerative disease, subacute sclerosing panencephalitis (SSPE).

- MMR is part of the UK immunization schedule, and over 5 million doses have been administered since 1988 when it was introduced.

- Measles vaccination rarely causes complications, including death in about 1 per million cases.

- Recently, concern has been expressed regarding a possible association between MMR vaccination and autism in children. Several large-scale epidemiological studies have found no evidence for such an association.

- There is not thought to be any risk of developing autism due to MMR vaccination.

- Giving measles, mumps and rubella vaccines separately inevitably reduces the uptake of these vaccines, increases the time for which children can contract these diseases, and exposes them to the trauma of six extra injections. Some parts of London where the vaccination rate has fallen below 70 per cent are facing a measles epidemic.

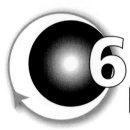

Respiratory problems

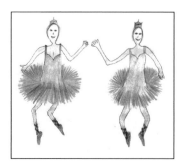

? Questions for each of the clinical cases

Q1: What is the likely differential diagnosis?
Q2: What issues in the given history support the diagnosis?
Q3: What additional features in the history would you seek to support a particular diagnosis?
Q4: What clinical examination would you perform, and why?
Q5: What investigations would be most helpful, and why?
Q6: What treatment options are appropriate?

Clinical cases

● CASE 6.1 – My 6-month-old baby has developed a cough and noisy breathing.

A 6-month-old baby has had a slight cold. Over the past day she has developed a mild temperature, worsening cough and wheezing.

● CASE 6.2 – My 4-year-old daughter has developed acute breathing difficulties with cough and wheezing.

A 4-year-old girl has developed wheeze and acute shortness of breath. She has mild eczema, and her brother needs an inhaler.

● CASE 6.3 – My 11-year-old son with cystic fibrosis has developed shortness of breath and a cough.

An 11-year-old boy who was diagnosed with cystic fibrosis as a neonate has increasing cough and dyspnoea. He has a temperature and is producing more sputum.

OCSE counselling cases 65

👥 OSCE counselling cases

OSCE COUNSELLING CASE 6.1 – My baby is always wheezy with a cough and cold. Does this mean she has asthma?

OSCE COUNSELLING CASE 6.2 – My son has been diagnosed with cystic fibrosis, what does this mean for him?

🔑 Key concepts

In order to work through the core clinical cases in this chapter, you will need to understand the following key concepts.

Airway inflammation and bronchoconstriction

- Inflammation of the lining of the small airway can cause swelling which reduces the size of the airway, making breathing more difficult.

- Bronchoconstriction or bronchospasm is a reversible narrowing of the small airways (bronchioles) in the lung which occurs as a result of contraction of the muscles surrounding the airway.

- Airway inflammation can occur as a result of inhaled allergens (such as pollen, house dust mite) or from viral infections (such as respiratory syncytial virus [q.v.] and influenza virus).

- Bronchoconstriction can be triggered by various factors, including exercise, cold air, smoke and dust.

- Both airway inflammation and bronchoconstriction can occur singly or in combination, and can cause shortness of breath, cough and wheeze.

- Wheezing in infancy is very common, and about 50 per cent will experience some wheezing, particularly after viral respiratory infections. Not all of these wheezy infants will develop asthma, and two-thirds of children who have wheeze under 3 years of age will be wheeze-free at 9 years.

Stridor

- A harsh, vibratory noise which occurs during the phases of breathing. Stridor can occur during inspiration, expiration or both (biphasic). *trachea + ul*

- Stridor is a sign of upper airway obstruction, and may be either acute or chronic. *a congenital ab of the laryngeal cartilage*

- Stridor from birth is usually due to a malformation at, or around, the larynx (e.g. laryngomalacia).

- The commonest cause of acute-onset stridor is viral croup (laryngotracheobronchitis), which usually affects children aged from 3 months to 5 years.

- Mild croup usually manifests as a barking cough (sounding like a seal). Common viruses associated with croup are parainfluenza virus (accounting for most cases), adenovirus, respiratory syncytial virus (q.v.), influenza and measles (q.v.).

- Viral croup is usually mild, and often can be alleviated by breathing moist or cool air. More severe cases respond to nebulized adrenaline and corticosteroids.

- Acute-onset stridor in a previously well child (particularly those over 1 year of age) should always raise the suspicion of an inhaled foreign body.

- Acute epiglottitis can cause severe, life-threatening stridor, but the incidence of this has fallen dramatically since the introduction of *Haemophilus influenza* type B vaccine (q.v.).

Bronchiolitis

- Bronchiolitis is a common lower respiratory tract viral infection affecting children under 2 years of age (peak age 3–6 months). It involves inflammation of the lower airway, resulting in breathing difficulties.

- Bronchiolitis is seasonal, and occurs mainly in the winter months.

- Initial symptoms are similar to the common cold with congestion, runny nose and mild cough and fever. These symptoms last for a day or two, and are followed by increasing breathing difficulty characterized by wheezing, worsening cough, tachypnoea and dyspnoea with sternal and/or subcostal recession (in-drawing of the chest with each breath).

- In mild cases, symptoms last 1–3 days. In severe cases, symptoms may progress more rapidly and include poor feeding and the development of respiratory failure and/or apnoea.

- A chest X-ray usually reveals hyperinflation and occasionally lobar infiltrates and/or atelectasis. Mostly the clinical illness is mild with an uneventful recovery in 5–7 days, though coughing may persist for up to 2 weeks.

- Hospitalization may be necessary, and a small proportion of infants may need respiratory support. At greatest risk are those with predisposing illness such as congenital heart disease or premature babies (particularly those with chronic lung disease).

- Respiratory syncytial virus (RSV) is the most commonly isolated agent in children aged less than 2 years and hospitalized for bronchiolitis. Other agents that cause bronchiolitis include influenza and parainfluenza viruses and adenoviruses.

- Treatment is mainly supportive – adequate hydration, oxygen if necessary. Monoclonal antibody prophylaxis and a specific antiviral agent may be of use in high-risk infants.

- RSV is highly contagious, and so strict measures to prevent cross-infection in hospitals are vital.

Asthma

- Asthma is a chronic inflammatory disorder of the airways. The inflammation usually results in widespread (but variable) airway obstruction and an increase in airway response to various stimuli.

- Asthma is one of the commonest chronic illnesses in childhood, affecting up to 15 per cent of schoolchildren.

- The typical inflammatory response is characterized by mucosal oedema, increased mucus production and contraction of bronchial muscles (bronchoconstriction).

- Asthma attacks can be precipitated by various triggers, including respiratory infections, allergic responses (e.g. to pollen, dust, animal dander), exercise, cold air and cigarette smoke.

- Symptoms include cough (particularly at night), breathlessness, chest tightness and wheeze.

- Clinical signs include wheeze on chest auscultation, chest wall recession and reduced peak expiratory flow rate (PEFR).

- Treatment includes avoidance of precipitating factors, short-acting bronchodilators (e.g. β_2 agonists) for mild disease; inhaled steroid prophylaxis, long-acting β_2 agonists and leukotriene antagonists can be used in more severe disease.

Cystic fibrosis

- Cystic fibrosis (CF) is an inherited condition which affects the lungs and digestion.

- CF is the commonest inherited condition in white Caucasians, with an incidence in this group of 1 in 2500 live births (carrier rate is 1 in 25). It is much less common in other ethnic groups.

- A defective gene causes an alteration of the movement of sodium chloride across the membranes of certain cells. This causes the lungs to produce thick, sticky mucus which blocks the small airways of the lungs, causing breathing difficulties and predisposing the lungs to infection. Thick secretions also block the enzymes which are normally produced by the pancreas to aid digestion. The reproductive system can also be affected, and this results in sterility.

- The commonest gene for CF (ΔF508) is found on chromosome 7. This accounts for about 80 per cent of UK CF patients, but over 800 mutations have been discovered.

- Symptoms include chronic, recurrent chest infections, poor absorption of fats from the diet which leads to fatty stools (steatorrhoea), and failure to thrive. About 10–20 per cent of infants with CF will present in the newborn period with meconium ileus, in which failure to pass thick tenacious meconium leads to intestinal obstruction.

- Treatment involves clearing the mucus from the lungs by means of postural drainage and chest physiotherapy. Chest infections are prevented by prophylactic antibiotics, and exacerbations of infections are treated aggressively with intravenous antibiotics. Dietary supplements are necessary to allow adequate absorption of food (pancreatic enzyme supplementation).

- The condition can be diagnosed before birth if the defective gene has been isolated from a previously diagnosed affected sibling.

- Treatment is lifelong, and at present no cure is available. Life expectancy is reduced, mainly as a consequence of strain on the heart from the chronic lung damage (cor pulmonale), and heart–lung transplantation may be the only option. However, adults with CF are surviving longer as treatment regimes improve.

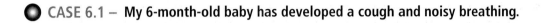

Answers

● CASE 6.1 – **My 6-month-old baby has developed a cough and noisy breathing.**

 Q1: What is the likely differential diagnosis?

A1

● Viral upper respiratory tract infection (URTI).

● Laryngotracheobronchitis (croup).

● Bronchiolitis; viral lower respiratory tract infection (LRTI).

● Milk aspiration.

● Bacterial pneumonia.

● Cardiac failure.

● Pertussis (whooping cough).

 Q2: What issues in the given history support the diagnosis?

A2

The baby has had coryzal symptoms prior to becoming unwell. Wheeze suggests lower respiratory tract involvement. The baby is at the peak age for bronchiolitis.

 Q3: What additional features in the history would you seek to support a particular diagnosis?

A3

● Has the illness steadily worsened, or was there a sudden deterioration? (as in aspiration).

● Ask about feeding and episodes of choking or coughing with feeds.

● Has the baby turned blue or stopped breathing?

● Have other family members (especially siblings) had similar symptoms? (spread of infection).

● Past medical history of heart or lung disease, prematurity, immunocompromise.

● Immunization history, including pertussis and RSV monoclonal antibody treatment.

Q4: What clinical examination would you perform, and why?

A4

- Check temperature, heart rate and respiratory rate.

- Assess cyanosis (check oxygen saturations), tracheal, sternal or subcostal recession (all of which would suggest severe respiratory distress).

- Auscultation of chest (wheezes ± crackles or stridor).

- Abdominal palpation (hepatomegaly may occur in heart failure).

Q5: What investigations would be most helpful, and why?

A5

- Nasopharyngeal aspirate for viral culture/immunofluorescence (RSV).

- Consider per nasal swab (for *Bordetella pertussis*).

- Consider a chest X-ray.

Q6: What treatment options are appropriate?

A6

- Fluid replacement – either by nasogastric tube or intravenous infusion if feeds not tolerated.

- Oxygen. If cyanosis or low oxygen saturations occur (aim to keep oxygen saturations >94%).

- Blood gases. If respiratory failure suspected.

- Respiratory support. If respiratory failure occurs.

- Anti-viral agents. Only in high-risk cases.

CASE 6.2 – My 4-year-old daughter has developed acute breathing difficulties with cough and wheezing.

Q1: What is the likely differential diagnosis?

A1

- Asthma.

- Inhaled foreign body.

- Viral LRTI.

- Bacterial LRTI.

- Pneumothorax.

Q2: What issues in the given history support the diagnosis?

A2

The symptoms are suggestive of asthma; there is a history of atopy and a family history of respiratory problems.

 Q3: What additional features in the history would you seek to support a particular diagnosis?

A3

- Ask about onset – sudden or gradual and associated symptoms, e.g. coryza, fever.
- Ask about small toys, nuts, etc. in the mouth (foreign body inhalation).
- Previous history of wheeze in infancy or nocturnal cough.
- Enquire further about family history of asthma or atopy. Exposure to potential precipitating factors – cold air, exercise, dust, animal dander, etc.

 Q4: What clinical examination would you perform, and why?

A4

- Temperature, heart rate (? tachycardia) and respiratory rate (? tachypnoea).
- Assess degree of respiratory difficulty – use of accessory muscles of respiration, intercostal and sub-costal recession, cyanosis (check oxygen saturations), ability to talk – cyanosis and inability to talk suggest severe respiratory compromise.
- Auscultation of the chest – widespread inspiratory and expiratory wheezes? A silent chest, in which the breath sounds are difficult to hear, suggests very poor air movement in the lungs and therefore severe respiratory compromise.

Q5: What investigations would be most helpful, and why?

A5

- Measurement of peak expiratory flow rate (PEFR) is important in older children, but children aged under 6 years are unlikely to be able to use the peak flow meter effectively.
- Blood gases and chest radiographs are rarely required.

 Q6: What treatment options are appropriate?

A6

- Inhaled β_2 agonist via spacer device or nebulizer.
- Inhaled ipratropium bromide.

- Oxygen (if O_2 saturations < 92%).

- Oral corticosteroids (prednisolone).

- Consider continuous nebulized salbutamol, or intravenous aminophylline or intravenous salbutamol (in refractory or life-threatening attacks, which may need to be given in the ITU setting).

CASE 6.3 – My 11-year-old son with cystic fibrosis has developed shortness of breath and a cough.

 Q1: What is the likely differential diagnosis?

A1

- Acute LRTI.

- Pneumothorax.

 Q2: What issues in the given history support the diagnosis?

A2

- History of CF, fever, change in sputum production.

 Q3: What additional features in the history would you seek to support a particular diagnosis?

A3

- Ask about previous exacerbations, colonization with *Pseudomonas aeruginosa,* haemoptysis and severe dyspnoea.

Q4: What clinical examination would you perform, and why?

A4

- Temperature, check for clubbing (chronic suppuration), assess chest expansion and oxygen saturations. Auscultate for wheeze and crepitations.

- Check weight and nutritional status.

Q5: What investigations would be most helpful, and why?

A5

- Send sputum or cough swab for urgent microbiological analysis.

- If possible, check spirometry.

Q6: What treatment options are appropriate?

A6

- Inhaled bronchodilator therapy.

- Intravenous antibiotics as recommended by local CF centre.

- Increase in physiotherapy regime.

👥 OSCE counselling cases

OSCE COUNSELLING CASE 6.1 – My baby is always wheezy with a cough and cold. Does this mean she has asthma?

- Wheezing during the first few years of life is very common.

- Up to 50 per cent of all children will experience at least one attack of wheezing during that time, and this is often caused by lower respiratory tract infections (usually viral).

- As long as the baby remains centrally pink and continues to feed well, this will be a self-limiting problem and no specific treatment is necessary.

- Some babies with more severe wheeze may benefit from treatment with inhaled bronchodilator therapy (ipratropium bromide or β_2 agonists via a face mask and spacer device may be of benefit in the acute phase of the illness).

- The occurrence of wheezing in early childhood does not necessarily mean that this will predispose to asthma, and approximately two-thirds of these children will be wheeze-free by the age of 9 years.

OSCE COUNSELLING CASE 6.2 – My son has been diagnosed with cystic fibrosis, what does this mean for him?

- Cystic fibrosis (CF) is the commonest inherited condition in white Caucasians, and primarily affects the lungs and the digestive system.

- When a person has CF there is a problem with the movement of salt across the lining of certain important cells in the lungs, pancreas and reproductive system. This causes a build up of thick, sticky mucus which can block the tubes in these parts of the body, affecting how well they work.

- The consequences of this build up of mucus is that the small airways of the lungs can become blocked; this makes breathing difficult and the lungs more susceptible to infection. The blockage in the pancreas means that important enzymes, which are necessary to digest fats, cannot get into the intestines and so fats in the diet are poorly absorbed.

- Common symptoms include poor growth and fatty stools as a result of poor absorption of fats; cough, wheeze and chronic chest infections occur as a consequence of the mucus in the lungs. Sometimes, babies with CF will have difficulty passing stool from birth and have a blocked intestine which may require operation (meconium ileus). Blockages in the reproductive organs lead to sterility.

- There is no cure for this condition, and individuals with CF have a shorter life expectancy. However, developments in the management of CF have been made which reduce the incidence of complications and increase the quality of life significantly.

- The mainstay of treatment is chest physiotherapy and regular antibiotics to reduce infections and lung complications, and enzyme supplements which help to improve fat digestion. Acute exacerbations of chest infections are treated very promptly, usually with intravenous antibiotics.

- CF is an inherited condition, and the most common changes in the genetic material are now known. Both parents are 'carriers' for the disease (i.e. they do not have the disease themselves, but have the ability to pass it on to their children) There is a one in four risk of this occurring with each pregnancy. It is now possible to detect whether an unborn baby has the disease if the genetic defect of their brother or sister with CF is known.

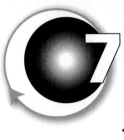

Fits, faints and funny turns

Questions

Clinical cases

Key concepts

Answers

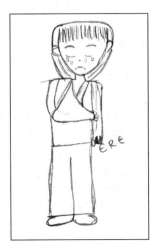

? **Questions for each of the clinical cases**

Q1: What is the likely differential diagnosis?
Q2: What issues in the given history support the given diagnosis?
Q3: What additional features in the given history would you seek to support a particular diagnosis?
Q4: What clinical examination would you perform, and why?
Q5: What investigations would be most helpful, and why?
Q6: What treatment options are appropriate?

Clinical cases

● CASE 7.1 – My newborn baby is going blue.

After a normal birth and delivery, my baby is now 12 hours old and has blue lips and tongue.

● CASE 7.2 – My 3-day-old baby has had a fit.

She was a healthy term infant who is breast-fed. She has a nasty infected umbilical cord stump.

● CASE 7.3 – My teenage son has just had a fit.

He stayed with friends at the weekend, and was found shaking all over this morning. He had a similar episode 3 months ago.

♟♟ OSCE counselling cases

OSCE COUNSELLING CASE 7.1 – My infant child has had his first febrile convulsion, what does it mean?

OSCE COUNSELLING CASE 7.2 – My toddler keeps having frightening breath-holding attacks.

🔑 Key concepts

In order to work through the core clinical cases in this chapter, you will need to understand the following key concepts.

Definitions

- A convulsion, seizure or fit is a neuronal motor discharge of all or part of the body, with one or more of the following elements: tonic or dystonic spasms (stiffening); clonic or myoclonic spasms (jerking); astatic episodes (falling).

- An epileptic fit or seizure consists of intermittent or stereotyped disturbance of cerebral cortical function, which may include any or all of the following abnormalities: motor; sensory; autonomic; emotional; behavioural; cognitive.

- Simple syncope or vaso-vagal attacks (faint) consist of a loss of consciousness, usually preceded by a drop in peripheral vascular resistance and blood pressure, together with bradycardia, and are self-limiting. This may be followed by a stiffening or reflex epileptic seizure.

- Breath-holding attacks or blue breath-holding is the end expiratory apnoea that commonly accompanies distraught crying in toddlers. It is the silent spell before the next loud inspiratory gasp and subsequent cry. These may also be followed by a spasm or reflex epileptic seizure.

- Febrile convulsion is a convulsion associated with fever (see below).

- Reflex anoxic syncope or reflex anoxic seizure is a massive vagal bradycardia leading to transient asystole which is 5–30 seconds in duration. The trigger may be a surprise or sudden pain. Because there is asystole and no circulation, the child is white and appears to be dead. These seizures are very frightening, may go on for years, and often no trigger is identified.

- Jitters are faster than convulsive twitches (faster than three per second), occur in response to an external stimulus, and can be stilled by touching the limb.

The purpose of electroencephalography (EEG)

- Electroencephalography is the most commonly requested neurological test.

- The electrical activity of the brain is recorded on paper in a number of channels (8 or 16).

- Rhythms are described in terms of frequency, e.g. slow waves of 0.5–3 Hz.

- EEG is indicated to clarify the type of epilepsy, once a clinical diagnosis of epilepsy has been made.

- Common patterns include a 3 per second spike and wave discharge in typical absence epilepsy; hypsarrhythmia in infantile spasms; burst suppression and slow waves with encephalopathy.

Neonatal seizures

- These are seizures occurring in the neonatal period; they usually have a cause.

- Causes include perinatal trauma, infection and metabolic abnormalities (e.g. hypoglycaemia, hypocalcaemia).

- Fits in neonates may present as cyanotic episodes or apnoeas, cycling limb movements or mouthing.

Idiopathic epilepsy

- These are seizures in infancy and childhood, without an obvious precipitating cause.

- These are classified by clinical features: (i) generalized (tonic-clonic, typical absence seizures, myoclonic and temporal; (ii) focal (e.g. focal sensory and focal motor seizures).

- However, fits are seldom classically tonic-clonic in type, and may easily be missed.

Cyanotic and acyanotic congenital heart disease

- Most heart disease in children is congenital.

- 6–8 per 1000 live births have significant cardiac malformations.

- Acyanotic heart lesions are not usually duct-dependent; that is, they may not rely on blood flow through the patent ductus arteriosus, which closes soon after birth. Examples include ventricular septal defect and atrial septal defect. The exceptions include critical aortic stenosis and coarctation of the aorta, which may be duct-dependent.

- Cyanotic heart lesions are duct-dependent, and so present with central cyanosis soon after birth. Examples include transposition of the great arteries, Ebstein's anomaly and tetralogy of Fallot.

- Peripheral cyanosis (blueness of the hands and feet) may occur when a child is cold or crying or ill from any cause.

- Central cyanosis is blueness of the tongue and lips, associated with a fall in arterial oxygen tension. It is seen clinically if the concentration of reduced haemoglobin in the blood is at least 5 g/dL, so may be difficult to spot in an anaemic child.

Answers

⬤ **CASE 7.1 – My newborn baby is going blue.**

 Q1: What is the likely differential diagnosis?

A1

- Cyanotic congenital heart disease, either from reduced pulmonary blood flow, or abnormal mixing of systemic venous and pulmonary venous blood.

- Persistent fetal circulation.

- Respiratory causes, e.g. pneumonia, aspiration, transient tachypnoea of the newborn, surfactant deficiency (respiratory distress syndrome), congenital abnormality.

- Shock, such as blood loss, beta-haemolytic streptococcal septicaemia.

- Hypothermia.

 Q2: What issues in the given history support the diagnosis?

A2

A diagnosis of cyanotic congenital heart disease would be supported by:

- Central cyanosis (of the lips and tongue) as opposed to peripheral cyanosis (hands and feet).

- Otherwise well infant or baby.

- Usually lack of respiratory distress unless co-existing respiratory disease (see above) or polycythaemia.

Q3: What additional features in the history would you seek to support a particular diagnosis?

A3

- Ask about antenatal scans: many hospitals undertake a four-chamber view of the heart at around 20 weeks.

- Does the infant get breathless on feeding? Any respiratory distress?

- Ask if the infant ever looked pink.

- Is there a family history of congenital heart disease?

Q4: What clinical examination would you perform, and why?

A4

- Check for central or peripheral cyanosis.

- Measure temperature.

- Examine for signs of shock, e.g. delayed capillary return, rapid thready pulse, pallor.

- Are there any other signs of systemic illness, e.g. hepatomegaly or rashes.

- Are there any dysmorphic features, e.g. Down's syndrome? (associated with increased incidence of congenital heart lesions)

- Check the pulses for brachio-brachial or brachio-femoral delay (coarctation of the aorta).

- Is there an audible heart murmur or palpable thrill?

 Q5: What investigations would be most helpful, and why?

A5

- Measure oxygen saturation in right hand and lower limb (pre- and post-ductal blood). Normal arterial oxygen saturation should be above 95 per cent. In cyanotic heart disease this can fall to the saturation of venous blood, i.e. <75 per cent.

- Nitrogen washout test. Place the infant in 100 per cent oxygen for 10 minutes. If the right radial SaO_2 is <15 kPa after this time, it makes a respiratory cause for cyanosis much less likely, and a diagnosis of cyanotic congenital heart disease is more likely.

- Perform chest X-ray. Look for signs of an abnormal heart outline and/or oligaemic or plethoric lung fields (congenital heart disease).

- ECG.

Q6: What treatment options are appropriate?

A6

- In duct-dependent lesions, give a prostaglandin (PGE_2) infusion. This is to maintain the patency of the ductus arteriosus to allow mixing of venous and arterial blood.

- Refer to a specialist paediatric cardiology unit for echocardiography and definitive diagnosis.

- Definitive surgical treatment depends on the nature of the lesion. Some lesions are correctable surgically (e.g. transposition of the great arteries); others are more complex, and may not be correctable.

● CASE 7.2 – **My 3-day-old baby has had a fit.**

Q1: What is the likely differential diagnosis?

A1

Most fits in infants have an identifiable cause, as opposed to fits in older children, which are usually idiopathic.

- Consider meningitis: this is usually associated with septicaemia in the first week.

- Low serum levels of calcium, magnesium or sodium can all cause fits.

- Drug withdrawal, for instance maternal opiate abuse in pregnancy.

- Inborn errors of metabolism, such as organic acidaemias.

- Fitting in the first 48 hours of life is most commonly due to perinatal hypoxia/ischaemia, intracranial trauma or haemorrhage.

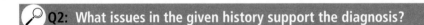

Q2: What issues in the given history support the diagnosis?

A2

- The infected stump suggests infection but this may be coincidental.

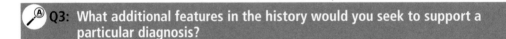

Q3: What additional features in the history would you seek to support a particular diagnosis?

A3

- Was there a history of difficult labour, i.e. prolonged, forceps (perinatal hypoxia, intracranial trauma)?

- Was there prolonged rupture of the membranes (sepsis)?

- Was there a maternal history of drug abuse (drug withdrawal)?

- Is there a family history of stillbirths or neonatal deaths (some inborn errors)?

- Poor feeding.

Q4: What clinical examination would you perform, and why?

A4

- Examine the baby for signs of infection. A flare around or from the umbilicus would suggest a bacterial infection.

- Examine for signs of poor perfusion, e.g. sunken fontanelle, slow capillary refill and birth trauma (e.g. bruising, fractures).

- Observe conscious level and spontaneous movement. Is the baby irritable or drowsy?

- Tense fontanelle may suggest meningitis.
- If possible, observe and describe the fit.

 Q5: What investigations would be most helpful, and why?

A5

- Culture skin swabs, blood and CSF for infection.
- Consider a cranial ultrasound for evidence of intracranial haemorrhage.
- Check blood glucose, serum electrolytes, calcium and magnesium.

 Q6: What treatment options are appropriate?

A6

- Treat infection with systemic antibiotics.
- Suppress convulsions with anticonvulsants (phenobarbitone, phenytoin – but not diazepam as it may cause respiratory depression).
- Counsel the parents as to the cause.

● CASE 7.3 – My teenage son has just had a fit.

 Q1: What is the likely differential diagnosis?

A1

- Idiopathic epilepsy
- Syncope-related reflex epileptic seizure.
- Drug intoxication, e.g. alcohol.
- Hypoglycaemic episode, possibly secondary to alcohol.
- Trauma.
- Space-occupying intracranial lesion.

 Q2: What issues in the given history support the diagnosis?

A2

- Most fits in teenagers are idiopathic, as opposed to fits in infants, which usually have a cause.

- The previous episode of a fit makes the diagnosis of epilepsy more likely, and this is unlikely to be simple syncope.

- The history of shaking all over would be compatible with a generalized tonic–clonic seizure.

 Q3: What additional features in the history would you seek to support a particular diagnosis?

A3

- Get a detailed description of the episode from his friends.

- Was the son drinking with friends, or taking drugs?

- Has there been a preceding history of headaches or visual disturbance? (intracranial lesion).

- Does he regularly feel faint first thing in the morning? (hypoglycaemia, cortisol insufficiency, postural hypotension).

- Has he had a recent head injury, perhaps sports-related?

 Q4: What clinical examination would you perform, and why?

A4

- Look for signs of trauma.

- Pale, clammy, with a bradycardia would suggest a faint.

- Drowsiness, incontinence and reduced reflexes indicate a seizure.

- Pin-point pupils may suggest drug-taking.

- Fundoscopy (for optic disc swelling), reflexes, full neurological examination.

 Q5: What investigations would be most helpful, and why?

A5

- Check capillary blood glucose for hypoglycaemia.

- Consider blood or urine samples for drug levels if drug-taking is considered.

- Check blood pressure, both lying and standing. EEG to diagnose idiopathic epilepsy. Try to classify the seizure type.

Q6: What treatment options are appropriate?

A6

- Epilepsy should be treated with anticonvulsants (e.g. sodium valproate).

- The patient should be advised to carry a medic-alert bracelet or card with the diagnosis.

- The patient should be encouraged to inform his close relatives and work colleagues.

- Advice should be given regarding occupations (e.g. driving heavy goods vehicles), and sporting activities such as swimming.

⚖ OSCE counselling cases

OSCE COUNSELLING CASE 7.1 – My infant child has had his first febrile convulsion, what does it mean?

- Febrile convulsions are common, and affect about 3 per cent of all children.

- The commonest ages to be affected are between 6 months and 6 years.

- The convulsions are usually brief, lasting under 5 minutes, and generalized tonic–clonic.

- The precipitant is commonly a viral upper respiratory tract infection, with the convulsion occurring when the temperature is rising rapidly.

- Febrile convulsions often run in families.

- In about 15 per cent of cases, another febrile convulsion will occur during the same episode of illness.

- The risk of a further febrile convulsion with another illness is about 30 per cent.

- This does not mean your child will have epilepsy; the risk for epilepsy after febrile convulsion is only about 2–4 per cent.

- The immediate management is to make sure your child is safe and breathing. Use simple measures to reduce the temperature, e.g. anti-pyretic medication (paracetamol).

- Do not place anything in your child's mouth.

- Call an ambulance if; the convulsion is atypical (i.e. prolonged more than 5 minutes), one-sided, your child has a rash, or if your child goes blue.

OSCE COUNSELLING CASE 7.2 – My toddler keeps having frightening breath-holding attacks.

- Blue breath-holding attacks are common and benign. They occur when your child breathes out and pauses before breathing back in.

- They can be set off by crying, upset, pain.

- Your child may go blue and lose consciousness, but will rapidly recover.

- No drug treatment is necessary, although these episodes have been linked to iron deficiency and it would be worth checking your child is not anaemic.

- Attacks will resolve by themselves, but behaviour modification therapy with avoidance of confrontation may help.

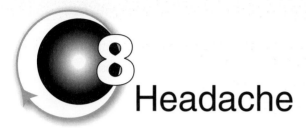

Headache

Questions

Clinical cases

Key concepts

Answers

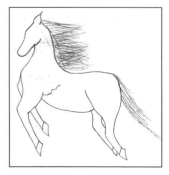

? **Questions for each of the clinical cases**

Q1: What is the likely differential diagnosis?
Q2: What issues in the given history support the diagnosis?
Q3: What additional features in the history would you seek to support a particular diagnosis?
Q4: What clinical examination would you perform, and why?
Q5: What investigations would be most helpful, and why?
Q6: What treatment options are appropriate?

Clinical cases

● **CASE 8.1 – My 8-year-old daughter has started to get headaches and is missing school.**

An 8-year-old girl has started to get recurrent symmetrical headaches. They are of gradual onset and are described thus '… like a band around my head'. She is having problems coping with the demands made by her school and has missed a third of her schooling this term.

● **CASE 8.2 – My 11-year-old son is having recurrent headaches with vomiting.**

An 11-year-old boy is having recurrent headaches which are throbbing, over his left eye, and associated with a visual aura. They are worsening in severity and frequency, but his school progress is good. His mother gets migraines that respond to treatment with triptans.

● **CASE 8.3 – My 6-year-old girl has a headache and has gone off her legs.**

A 6-year-old child presents with a 4-week history of a constant progressive headache which makes her cry inconsolably, with a week's history of an unsteady gait and slurred speech.

OSCE counselling cases

OSCE COUNSELLING CASE 8.1 – **My 11-year-old son has migraine.**

OSCE COUNSELLING CASE 8.2 – **My 6-year-old girl needs a CT head scan.**

🔑 Key concepts

In order to work through the core clinical cases in this chapter, you will need to understand the following key concepts.

Headache

- Headache is common in school children and young people. Some 95 per cent of schoolchildren report one headache per year.

- Headache is uncommon in preschool children.

The following classification of headache is useful in diagnosis:

- Acute

  - Febrile illness of any cause.

  - Acute sinusitis.

  - Intracranial sepsis (meningitis, encephalitis, abscess).

  - Head injury.

  - Space-occupying lesion.

  - Intracranial bleed.

  - Hypertension.

- Recurrent

  - Tension headache.

  - Migraine.

  - Ocular headaches due to refractive errors.

  - Space-occupying lesion.

  - Raised intracranial pressure.

  - Hypertension.

  - Poisoning, e.g. drug abuse, carbon monoxide (q.v.).

  - Seizures (q.v.).

Answers

 CASE 8.1 – My 8-year-old daughter has started to get headaches and is missing school.

 Q1: What is the likely differential diagnosis?

A1

- Tension headaches.
- Migraine.
- Raised intracranial pressure.
- Hypertension.
- Sinusitis.
- Benign intracranial hypertension.
- Carbon monoxide poisoning.

Q2: What issues in the given history support the diagnosis?

A2

The description of the headache as a 'band', its recurrent non-progressive nature, and the history of school problems suggest tension headaches.

Q3: What additional features in the history would you seek to support a particular diagnosis?

A3

Seek symptoms of:

- Migraine: aura, nausea, vomiting, pallor, focal neurology, abdominal pain, family history of migraine.
- Raised intracranial pressure: worsening school progress, behavioural change, early morning headaches, headaches at night, headaches worse on coughing, sneezing, laughing or bending over.

 Q4: What clinical examination would you perform, and why?

A4

- Plot height and weight.
- Measure blood pressure.

- Full neurological examination including conscious level, mentation, cranial nerves, e.g. visual fields in craniopharyngioma, other cranial nerve abnormalities in brainstem tumours, fundoscopy for papilloedema, cerebellar signs and cranial bruits, e.g. in arteriovenous malformations.

Q5: What investigations would be most helpful, and why?

A5

Investigations are only conducted if indicated by clinical assessment. A diagnosis can often be made without investigation. Urgent cranial imaging (CT scan or MRI scan) is indicated if there is evidence of:

- Altered consciousness.
- Focal neurological signs.
- Hypertension.
- Papilloedema.
- Headaches worsening (e.g. waking at night).
- Change in behaviour or personality.
- Worsening school performance.

Q6: What treatment options are appropriate?

A6

Tension headaches require reassurance and analgesia. School issues need to be addressed by working with the school doctor and relevant teachers.

CASE 8.2 – My 11-year-old son is getting recurrent headaches with vomiting.

Q1: What is the likely differential diagnosis?

A1

- Migraine.
- Tension headaches.
- Raised intracranial pressure.
- Hypertension.
- Sinusitis.
- Benign intracranial hypertension.
- Carbon monoxide poisoning (q.v.).

Q2: What issues in the given history support the diagnosis?

A2

- Recurrent headaches associated with nausea, an aura and a family history are suggestive of migraine.
- Some 50 per cent of children with migraine have a first-degree relative with the same diagnosis.

 Q3: What additional features in the history would you seek to support a particular diagnosis?

A3

Seek details of:

- Amount of school missed.
- Duration of each headache.
- Severity.
- Triggers.
- Treatment given so far.
- Behaviour or personality change.
- Nocturnal headache.

 Q4: What clinical examination would you perform, and why?

A4

- Measure blood pressure.
- Full neurological examination including conscious level, mentation, cranial nerves, fundoscopy, cranial bruits and cerebellar signs.

 Q5: What investigations would be most helpful, and why?

A5

- Investigations are only conducted if indicated by clinical assessment.
- A diagnosis can often be made without investigation.
- Indications for urgent cranial imaging are listed in Case 8.1, A5.

Q6: What treatment options are appropriate?

A6

Management of migraine includes:

- Diagnosis and explanation of cause.

- Identification of triggers through a headache diary.

- Avoidance of triggers.

- Prompt treatment of early symptoms with analgesia such as paracetamol, which may be combined with an anti-emetic.

- Discussion about the pros of prophylaxis (reduced frequency of headaches) versus the cons (need to take medication daily, side effects such as tiredness).

- Triptans have not been used extensively in children, and are not licensed for this age group.

● **CASE 8.3 – My 6-year-old girl has a headache and has gone off her legs.**

 Q1: What is the likely differential diagnosis?

A1

- Brain tumour.

- Intracranial infection, e.g. brain abscess, meningitis, septicaemia, encephalitis.

- Trauma with intracranial injury.

- Carbon monoxide poisoning (q.v.).

 Q2: What issues in the given history support the diagnosis?

A2

The recent onset of a severe, progressive headache associated with focal neurological signs suggests intracranial pathology.

 Q3: What additional features in the history would you seek to support a particular diagnosis?

A3

Seek a history of:

- Previous episodes.

- Fever.

- Onset of headache.

- Behaviour and personality change.

- School progress.

- Contact with infectious diseases, travel (e.g. malaria).

- Family history of migraine.

 Q4: What clinical examination would you perform, and why?

A4

- Measure blood pressure.

- Examine skin for neurocutaneous signs (e.g. neurofibromas, café au lait spots in neurofibromatosis).

- Full neurological examination including conscious level, mentation, cranial nerves, fundoscopy, cranial bruits and cerebellar signs.

 Q5: What investigations would be most helpful, and why?

A5

- Urgent intracranial imaging (CT head or MRI).

Further investigations as indicted by clinical assessment and imaging:

- Full blood count: a raised white cell count suggest infection.

- Thick film for malaria parasites (q.v.): if history of foreign travel.

- Urea and electrolytes: for syndrome of inappropriate ADH (SIADH).

- Carbon monoxide levels: if history of contact.

- Lead levels.

Q6: What treatment options are appropriate?

A6

- Rapid clinical assessment may indicate need for urgent intervention before a detailed history can be taken. Basic and advanced life support should be instituted as required.

- Intravenous antibiotics and antivirals.

- Management of raised intracranial pressure.

- Urgent referral for neurosurgical opinion.

👥 OSCE counselling cases

OSCE COUNSELLING CASE 8.1 – My 11-year-old son has migraine.

An 11-year-old boy has recurrent headaches which are throbbing, over his left eye, and are associated with a visual aura. They are worsening in severity and frequency, but his school progress is good. His mother gets migraines that respond to treatment with triptans. Clinical assessment suggests that the boy also has migraine.

Families, children and young people with migraine require verbal and written information. They need to know:

- How their symptoms fit the diagnosis of migraine.

- Fear of 'brain tumour' is a common reason for presentation; your careful and thorough assessment has excluded this, and provided the reasons why.

- The cause of migraine is not known; one theory is that blood vessels in one part of the brain become narrowed when the sufferer gets altered sensations, then open wide so that may lead to the headache. The blood vessels then return to normal. The theory does not explain the whole story however, and chemicals in the brain may also play a part.

- Triggers are important in setting off migraine: diet (e.g. chocolate, cheese), environment (e.g. smoke, bright lights), medication (e.g. the pill), hormones (e.g. menstruation, anxiety). Sometimes, triggers can be identified and avoided by keeping a 'headache diary'.

- Prompt treatment of early symptoms with an analgesic such as paracetamol, which may be combined with an anti-emetic.

- Discussion about the pros of prophylaxis (reduced frequency of headaches) versus the cons (need to take medication daily, side effects such as tiredness).

OSCE COUNSELLING CASE 8.2 – My 6-year-old girl needs a CT head scan.

- CT scans create a detailed picture of the brain and the head.

- Usually, they are carried out on the same day, and you can go home on the same day as you have one.

- The scanner looks like a small tunnel.

- Sedation or a general anaesthetic may be needed if you are too young to lie still. MRI scanners are noisy and may frighten young children.

- In order to see certain parts of the brain, you may need to be given a small amount of dye which is harmless, but shows up on the pictures. The dye is given via a small needle which is inserted into a vein on the back of the child's hand. We will use a local anaesthetic cream to make sure that the needle injection is not painful.

- Play specialists should rehearse the procedure with children prior to the scan to ensure that they understand what will happen.

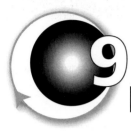

9 Diarrhoea and vomiting

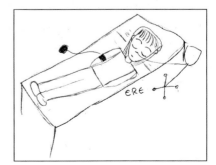

? Questions for each of the clinical cases

Q1: What is the likely differential diagnosis?
Q2: What issues in the given history support the given diagnosis?
Q3: What additional features in the given history would you seek to support a particular diagnosis?
Q4: What clinical examination would you perform, and why?
Q5: What investigations would be most helpful, and why?
Q6: What treatment options are appropriate?

Clinical cases

● CASE 9.1 – **My 6-month-old son started screaming with pain and drawing up his legs. There is nothing I can do to console him.**

A previously well child has developed sudden onset episodes of screaming and drawing up his legs; he has not opened his bowels recently, and looks very pale.

● CASE 9.2 – **My toddler has developed sickness and diarrhoea. Most of the other children at his nursery have developed it as well.**

A 14-month-old boy has started vomiting and has loose watery stools up to eight times a day. He has a slight fever and is rather quiet. Other mothers at the nursery report similar findings.

● CASE 9.3 – **My 4-week-old boy has suddenly started vomiting up all his feeds and can't stop, even though he still wants to feed.**

This baby was born at term after a normal pregnancy. He fed well initially, but recently he has been vomiting after every feed. Sometimes, the vomiting is forceful and shoots out of his mouth. He still seems hungry and feeds vigorously.

OSCE counselling cases

OSCE COUNSELLING CASE 9.1 – My child cries all the time with colic, what shall I do?

OSCE COUNSELLING CASE 9.2 – My baby keeps being sick after feeds, I am changing clothes all the time, what should I do?

🔑 Key concepts

In order to work through the core clinical cases in this chapter, you will need to understand the following key concepts.

Assessment of dehydration

Dehydration is assessed clinically. The symptoms and signs to look for include:

- Thirst, irritability, lethargy.
- Dry mucous membranes.
- Sunken eyes.
- Rapid, thready pulse.
- Sunken fontanelle (in babies).
- Reduced tissue turgor (this is a reduction in the elasticity of the skin).
- Reduced capillary return.
- Pallor and mottled extremities.
- Reduced urine output.
- Reduced level of consciousness (in severe cases).

Stool frequency and diarrhoea

- Newborn babies pass sticky black stools (meconium) after birth.
- Breast-fed babies pass frequent, loose, seedy yellow stools.
- Breast-fed infants may pass up to 8–10 stools a day. Bottle-fed babies usually pass stools less frequently (2–3 times a day).
- Stools that are watery or soak into the nappy with no solid material are abnormal.
- The presence of blood in the stool indicates pathology, e.g. infection, mucosal tear, gastrointestinal bleeding.
- Diarrhoea is the passage of frequent, loose stools.
- The causes of diarrhoea are acute (e.g. gastroenteritis, associated with antibiotic treatment) and chronic (e.g. post-infectious malabsorption, coeliac disease and inflammatory bowel disease).
- Treatment involves correction of any dehydration, and is then directed to the underlying cause.
- Note: Oral rehydration therapy consists of a glucose and electrolyte powder which is reconstituted with water. The principle is the linked active transport of sodium and glucose absorption in the small intestine. Glucose and sodium are co-transported across the intestinal mucosa with water.
- Give maintenance fluids plus replacement of deficit and ongoing losses. Aim to correct dehydration within 4–12 hours with 50–100 ml/kg oral rehydration fluid given as frequent small amounts.

Infantile colic

- This is very common in infancy, and consists of paroxysmal, inconsolable crying or screaming together with drawing up of the knees. This can occur several times a day, but it is more common in the evening.

- The cause is unknown, but is benign, and it is not associated with other disease. Indeed, it is not recognized in some countries.

- Babies are well between episodes.

- Management is by swaddling the child up for comfort, and cuddling.

- It resolves usually by 3 months of age.

Gastro-oesophageal reflux

- This is common in infancy, and ranges from the 'posset' of a mouthful of milk after a feed to vomiting up most of the feed. If severe it may lead to failure to thrive, anaemia, and aspiration pneumonitis.

- Most reflux resolves by 12 months of age.

- Complications can include oesophagitis causing pain, bleeding and anaemia; dystonic movements of the head and neck (Sandifer syndrome); apnoeas in preterm infants. It is more common in infants with cerebral palsy (q.v.).

- The cause is thought to be functional immaturity of the lower oesophageal sphincter, leading to inappropriate relaxation.

- Diagnosis is usually made by the history, although a contrast swallow or 24-hour oesophageal pH study may be indicated in more severe cases.

- Infants with mild uncomplicated reflux can be diagnosed clinically and managed with thickening agents added to the feeds.

- Sometimes, drugs which help to reduce acid in the stomach (e.g. ranitidine) or help bowel peristalsis may be necessary.

- The most severe cases are treated by fundoplication, where the stomach fundus is wrapped around the intra-abdominal oesophagus.

Intussusception

- This is the invagination of one segment of bowel into an adjacent lower segment, cutting off the blood supply to the invaginated segment as it progresses.

- It usually begins proximal to the ileocaecal valve.

- Intussusception is the commonest cause of bowel obstruction in infants after the neonatal period, occurring most commonly at the age of 6–9 months.

- It characteristically presents with paroxysmal, colicky abdominal pain and pallor. The infant draws up the legs with the pain.

- Vomiting and diarrhoea are common, and sometimes a sausage-shaped mass is palpable in the abdomen.

- Late presentations may include passage of 'redcurrant jelly' stools, which contain blood and mucus.

- It is possible that viral infection leads to swelling of Peyer's patches (lymph tissue in the small intestine) from which the intussusception may begin.

- An abdominal X-ray may show small bowel obstruction. Treatment is usually by reduction of the intussusception with air per rectum; alternatively contrast medium may be used.

- Profound shock may occur due to pooling of fluid in the gut. Intravenous fluids are usually required to prevent circulatory failure.

Pyloric stenosis

- Affects infants from 2–8 weeks of age, more frequently males, and first-born children.

- There may also be a family history, especially in the mother.

- The cause is hypertrophy of the pylorus muscle at the exit of the stomach.

- There is persistent uncontrollable vomiting which is not bile-stained.

- The vomiting is projectile, i.e. it shoots out with force.

- Vomiting usually occurs within 30 minutes of a feed, and the infant is hungry afterwards.

- The infant may be constipated and become dehydrated.

- A hypochloraemic alkalosis develops from vomiting the acid stomach contents. Some infants are mildly jaundiced.

- On examination, gastric peristalsis may be visible in the epigastrium following a feed.

- The diagnosis is made by palpation of an enlarged hard pylorus in the right upper quadrant during a test feed (see below). An ultrasound scan of the pyloric region may also be diagnostic.

- A test feed is performed as follows. Place the child on its mother's lap and allow to feed, while positioning yourself kneeling to the left side of the child's abdomen. Observe the abdomen for signs of peristalsis, particularly a wave occurring across the abdomen. Palpate using your left hand in the infant's right upper quadrant for a mass the size and consistency of the end of your nose.

- The management is to correct the dehydration and electrolyte imbalance, and undertake a pyloromyotomy: the pylorus is incised to divide the hypertrophied muscle fibres, but not the pyloric mucosa.

Answers

 CASE 9.1 – My 6-month-old son started screaming with pain and drawing up his legs.

 Q1: What is the likely differential diagnosis?

A1

- Acute infantile colic.

- Acute intussusception.

- Acute gastroenteritis.

- Testicular torsion (in boys).

- Strangulated inguinal hernia.

- Other cause of intestinal obstruction.

- Urinary tract infection.

- Non-accidental injury

- Serious bacterial illness of any cause, e.g. meningitis, septicaemia.

 Q2: What issues in the given history support the diagnosis?

A2

Acute intussusception is supported by the sudden onset of the condition in a previously well child, inconsolable pain, and drawing up of the legs. Infantile colic would have presented earlier and be intermittent, with the child completely well between episodes.

Q3: What additional features in the history would you seek to support a particular diagnosis?

A3

- Ask about any vomiting and diarrhoea which may occur in gastroenteritis and also intussusception.

- What colour are the stools? (i.e. is there blood present)

- Ask about pallor or any recent viral infection.

Q4: What clinical examination would you perform, and why?

A4

- Assess the level of dehydration and shock (acute circulatory failure).
- Examine the abdomen between bouts of pain for any tenderness or masses.
- Listen for bowel sounds (in intestinal obstruction bowel sounds are characteristically tinkling).
- Examine the hernial orifices and testes for erythema, tenderness or swelling.

 Q5: What investigations would be most helpful, and why?

A5

- Check a blood sample for acidosis, urea and electrolytes, and full blood count.
- A plain abdominal X-ray would assist in the diagnosis of obstruction.
- Urinalysis, blood culture, full blood count.

 Q6: What treatment options are appropriate?

A6

- If present, correct shock with intravenous fluids.
- Reduction of the intussusception with air insufflation under radiological control.
- An obstructed hernia will require urgent surgery.

CASE 9.2 – My toddler has developed sickness and diarrhoea, and most of the children at his nursery have developed it as well.

 Q1: What is the likely differential diagnosis?

A1

- Acute viral gastroenteritis.
- Bacterial gastroenteritis, e.g. *Salmonella, Campylobacter, Shigella* dysentery.
- Lactose intolerance.
- Coeliac disease.

Q2: What issues in the given history support the diagnosis?

A2

The presence of diarrhoea and vomiting in the child's nursery supports the diagnosis of an infective cause (e.g. rotavirus). This also makes food-borne infections a possibility.

 Q3: What additional features in the history would you seek to support a particular diagnosis?

A3

- Ask about the frequency of dirty nappies. Up to four dirty nappies a day is probably normal.
- Ask about the nature of the stools: profuse watery diarrhoea with little solid material suggests gastroenteritis. Ask if there is any blood in the stools or vomit.
- If the vomiting is bile-stained, consider obstruction.
- Ask about any foreign travel (bacterial gastroenteritis more likely).

 Q4: What clinical examination would you perform, and why?

A4

- Examine the abdomen.
- Assess the level of hydration.
  - Moderate (5%) dehydration gives the signs of irritability, dry lips and mouth, and eyes slightly sunken.
  - Severe (10%) dehydration is suggested by altered consciousness, rapid thready pulse, reduced skin turgor.

 Q5: What investigations would be most helpful, and why?

A5

- Consider checking serum sodium to look for hyponatraemic or hypernatraemic dehydration.
- Take a stool sample for culture and microscopy for ova, cysts and parasites, and immunofluorescence for rotavirus (the commonest cause of acute gastroenteritis in winter months).

 Q6: What treatment options are appropriate?

A6

- Oral rehydration therapy rather than intravenous fluid therapy.
- Reintroduce feeds as soon as possible when rehydrated. Do not stop breast feeding.

● **Case 9.3 – My 4-week-old boy has suddenly started vomiting all his feeds.**

 Q1: What is the likely differential diagnosis?

A1

- Pyloric stenosis.

- Acute gastroenteritis.

- Urinary tract infection.

- Gastro-oesophageal reflux.

- Neonatal intestinal obstruction (e.g. malrotation, Ladd's bands, duodenal web).

 Q2: What issues in the given history support the diagnosis?

A2

Pyloric stenosis is suggested by the timing of onset of vomiting (usually within 20 minutes of a feed); the age (2–8 weeks at presentation) and the desire to continue feeding, which is present in the early stages but is lost as the infant becomes dehydrated.

Q3: What additional features in the history would you seek to support a particular diagnosis?

A3

- Birth history, early feeding and time to pass meconium.

- Ask about any previous history of vomiting, particularly with feeds.

- Enquire about stool frequency.

- Is the child the first in the family and is there a family history of pyloric stenosis?

Q4: What clinical examination would you perform, and why?

A4

- Assess level of dehydration.

- Examine the infant's abdomen before, during and after a test feed (q.v.).

Q5: What investigations would be most helpful, and why?

A5

- An ultrasound of the abdomen is most helpful, to confirm the presence of pyloric hypertrophy.

- Check urea, electrolytes and chloride for evidence of dehydration and hypochloraemic metabolic alkalosis.

 Q6: What treatment options are appropriate?

A6

- Correction of the metabolic abnormalities with intravenous fluids, including potassium.

- Surgery: pyloromyotomy, only after correction of metabolic abnormalities.

👥 OSCE counselling cases

OSCE COUNSELLING CASE 9.1 – My child cries all the time with colic, what shall I do?

- Colic is very common, and affects almost all babies at some point; the cause is unknown.

- Colic is completely harmless and goes away by itself, usually by the age of 3 months.

- Proprietary remedies may help some, but not all, babies.

- Do not give alcohol in any form as the baby may go hypoglycaemic.

- Wrap the baby up well and cuddle him.

- If you just can't cope any longer, please seek help from family and friends, or your health visitor or GP.

OSCE COUNSELLING CASE 9.2 – My baby keeps being sick after feeds, I am changing clothes all the time, what should I do?

- Gastro-oesophageal reflux is common, and usually harmless.

- It is more inconvenient than anything else as it involves lots of washing and makes the house smell.

- It happens when food in the stomach gets pushed back up the gullet, due to immaturity of the muscle at the base of the gullet that should stop this reflux.

- The acid that comes up with the food may irritate the baby and cause discomfort.

- Simple measures may help: nurse the baby upright or at 30 degrees after feeds; try adding a proprietary thickener to bottle feeds.

- If necessary, there are drugs that will help.

- Please let the doctor know if there is blood in the refluxed milk.

- If it persists, further investigation and treatment may be necessary.

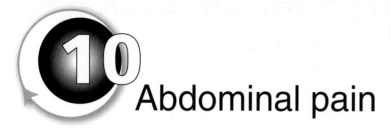

10 Abdominal pain

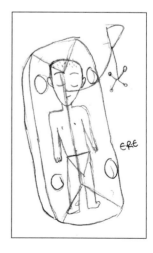

? **Questions for each of the clinical cases**

Q1: What is the likely differential diagnosis?
Q2: What issues in the given history support the diagnosis?
Q3: What additional features in the history would you seek to support a particular diagnosis?
Q4: What clinical examination would you perform, and why?
Q5: What investigations would be most helpful, and why?
Q6: What treatment options are appropriate?

Clinical cases

● Case 10.1 – My 8-year-old son has abdominal pain with smoky coloured urine.

An 8-year-old boy presents to his GP with acute abdominal pain. The pain is lower abdominal and constant. He has been off his food for about 10 days, and has lost some weight. There has been no vomiting. In addition, he recently had fever with a sore throat. His urine looks 'smoky' and red, as if there is blood in it.

● Case 10.2 – My 9-year-old daughter has been thirsty for days and passing lots of urine. Now she has tummy ache and is drowsy.

A 9-year-old girl had a viral illness a week ago and has recently been drinking a large glass of water every hour or so. She is passing a lot of urine, has to rush to the toilet, and wet the bed during the previous night. Over the past few hours she has been very sleepy, and her breath smells funny.

● Case 10.3 – My 13-month-old child is getting thinner, with frequent tummy aches and diarrhoea.

This child gained weight steadily during the first 6 months of life, but since then weight gain has slowed down. He looks pale and skinny, and passes frequent bulky stools which have an offensive smell.

👥 OSCE counselling cases

OSCE COUNSELLING CASE 10.1 – **My 7-year-old son keeps getting tummy ache on the way to school.**

OSCE COUNSELLING CASE 10.2 – **My 10-year-old daughter is constipated, and this is very distressing. Can you give her something?**

⚷ Key concepts

In order to work through the core clinical cases in this chapter, you will need to understand the following key concepts.

- Problems arising in the gastrointestinal system can produce a wide variety of symptoms, and are responsible for a high proportion of attendances at hospital accident and emergency departments.

- Many non-gastrointestinal disturbances can also cause abdominal pain.

- Abdominal pain is often non-specific, so it is important to keep an open mind regarding the cause until a firm diagnosis is reached.

- Medical causes of abdominal pain are common and include the following.

Acute post-streptococcal glomerulonephritis

- Acute nephritis in childhood is a recognized complication of a streptococcal sore throat. Other recognized complications include rheumatic fever and erythema marginatum.

- Glomerular inflammation limits glomerular blood flow and reduces glomerular filtration rate. This results in reduced urine output (oliguria) and volume overload. Other features include hypertension; peri-orbital oedema and haematuria with proteinuria.

- In the UK this is usually a mild illness, but it frequently causes abdominal pain.

- The outlook is good, symptoms usually resolve within 2 weeks.

Diabetic ketoacidosis

- Up to 45 per cent of children with type 1 diabetes will present with diabetic ketoacidosis.

- Insulin production is insufficient to maintain normoglycaemia, or to suppress lipase activity. Glucose is unable to enter cells, which consequently are starved of energy. Body metabolism is redirected from an anabolic to a catabolic state. Lipase breaks down fats to fatty acids and glycerol. Fatty acids enter the tricarboxylic acid cycle via acetoacetate, but are unable to progress be further metabolized due to a lack of reducing power (NADH), and so are diverted towards ketone production. This leads to ketoacidosis.

- The combination of dehydration and ketones is thought to be responsible for the acute abdominal pain which occurs frequently in diabetic ketoacidosis.

Coeliac disease

- This is an enteropathy (inflammation of the lining of the gut) where the gliadin fraction of gluten (found in wheat and wheat-based products) causes a damaging immunological response in the small intestinal mucosa.

- Villi become progressively shorter then absent, leading to a flat mucosa. This results in malabsorption and can be demonstrated on a jejunal biopsy.

- The prevalence of coeliac disease is about 1 in 3000, but this may be a considerable underestimate.

- Children usually present in the first 2 years of life with failure to thrive following the introduction of gluten to the diet.

- Symptoms include failure to thrive (weight faltering q.v.), irritability, loose and frequent stools, abdominal pain, and wasting of the buttocks.

- Complete exclusion of gluten in the diet should result in resolution of symptoms within months.

- Strict adherence to a gluten-free diet is also thought to reduce the long-term increased risk of bowel lymphoma.

- Children may undergo a follow-up biopsy to confirm that the villi have recovered. Nowadays, compliance with treatment is monitored with autoantibody titres.

Answers

 CASE 10.1 – My 8-year-old son has abdominal pain with smoky coloured urine.

Q1: What is the likely differential diagnosis?

A1

Causes of haematuria with abdominal pain include:

- Urinary tract infection.
- Trauma.
- Acute post streptococcal glomerulonephritis.
- Henoch–Schönlein purpura.
- Renal calculi.
- Haemolytic uraemic syndrome.
- Sickle cell disease.
- Wilms' tumour.
- Bleeding disorders.
- Bilharzia.

Q2: What issues in the given history support the diagnosis?

A2

- A diagnosis of urinary tract infection would be supported if there was a history of previous infections, or unexplained low-grade fever, or dysuria.
- Acute post-streptococcal glomerulonephritis would be supported by a history of sore throat in the previous 3 weeks.

Q3: What additional features in the history would you seek to support a particular diagnosis?

A3

Ask about lethargy, dysuria, reduced urine output, and peri-orbital oedema in the days preceding presentation.

Q4: What clinical examination would you perform, and why?

A4

- Measure blood pressure and compare to age-standardized charts. Hypertension would make the diagnosis of acute renal failure likely. Hypertension may also occur secondary to chronic renal failure associated with recurrent urinary tract infections.

- Examine the abdomen for tenderness and masses.

 Q5: What investigations would be most helpful, and why?

A5

- Examine the urine for protein, red cells and haemoglobinuria, and perform a stick test for nitrite (indicative of infection).

- Acute post-streptococcal glomerulonephritis is diagnosed by a raised Anti-Streptolysin O (ASO) titre and low complement C3 levels that return to normal after 2–3 weeks.

- Urea and electrolytes (these may show a raised urea and creatinine, and raised potassium in acute renal failure).

- Urine for microscopy, culture and sensitivity (to exclude urinary tract infection).

Q6: What treatment options are appropriate?

A6

- Urinary tract infections respond to appropriate antibiotics, depending on the sensitivity of the organism cultured.

- Acute post-streptococcal glomerulonephritis requires supportive management only. This includes monitoring fluid balance, blood pressure and renal function; salt and water restriction to avoid fluid overload; penicillin as prophylaxis against streptococcal infection; diuretics and anti-hypertensives to treat the sequelae of renal failure.

- Renal biopsy may be indicated only if the course of the disease is prolonged

- Dialysis may be required if renal failure and hypertension progress, or heart failure ensues.

 CASE 10.2 – My 9-year-old daughter has been thirsty for days and passing lots of urine.

Q1: What is the likely differential diagnosis?

A1

- Diabetic ketoacidosis.

- Mesenteric adenitis.

- Urinary tract infection, pyelonephritis.

- Acute post-streptococcal glomerulonephritis.
- Acute appendicitis.

 Q2: What issues in the given history support the diagnosis?

A2

- This child has a short prodromal illness, with weight loss. Diabetes at presentation can often be precipitated by a prodromal viral illness such as a sore throat.
- Other features include starting to wet the bed again after being dry at night (secondary enuresis), polydipsia and polyuria and funny-smelling breath (ketones, which smell like pear-drops).

Q3: What additional features in the history would you seek to support a particular diagnosis?

A3

- Ask about lethargy.
- Has there been any history of vaginal thrush? (due to fungal infection). Balanitis (inflammation of the glans penis) in boys?
- Is there a family history of diabetes? (present in about 10% of cases)

Q4: What clinical examination would you perform, and why?

A4

- Look for signs of abdominal tenderness and guarding (may be present in both diabetic ketoacidosis and acute appendicitis).
- Ketones on the breath (smells like pear drops).
- Examine for signs of dehydration (reduced skin turgor, dry mucous membranes, sunken eyes).
- Examine for signs of shock (reduced capillary refill time, rapid thready pulse, pallor, cool peripheries, altered consciousness).

 Q5: What investigations would be most helpful, and why?

A5

- Test the urine for glucose, ketones and nitrites.
- Venous glucose estimation.
- Check a capillary blood gas for metabolic acidosis.

Q6: What treatment options are appropriate?

A6

- Treat shock by restoring circulating blood volume. This involves intravenous administration of physiological (0.9%) saline.

- Rehydrate slowly with 0.9 per cent saline, by calculating the fluid deficit, maintenance requirement, and ongoing losses, and replace over 24–48 hours.

- Add potassium to the fluid used to rehydrate, as there is a total body deficit of potassium.

- Replace insulin via a continuous infusion initially, and then introduce a sliding scale when the blood glucose falls below 12 mmol/L.

- Change to subcutaneous insulin when the child is eating and drinking. This is usually in the form of a mixture of short- and intermediate-acting insulin given as one injection, twice a day.

● **CASE 10.3 – My 13-month-old child is getting thinner, with frequent tummy aches and diarrhoea.**

 Q1: What is the likely differential diagnosis?

A1

- Coeliac disease.

- Other causes of malabsorption such as inflammatory bowel disease, lactose intolerance, milk allergy and cows' milk protein intolerance.

- Feeding problems.

- Parasitic infestation.

- Malignancy such as Wilms' tumour, neuroblastoma in a younger child.

- Mesenteric tuberculosis.

 Q2: What issues in the given history support the diagnosis?

A2

- Acquired malabsorption such as coeliac disease may present with failure to thrive in a previously thriving child, so a history of getting thinner is not uncommon. Other causes include feeding problems, lactose intolerance and cows' milk protein intolerance.

- In coeliac disease, increased bowel frequency occurs; this is usually combined with urgency and loose stools.

Q3: What additional features in the history would you seek to support a particular diagnosis?

A3

- Ask about symptoms of allergy: rashes, wheeze, swelling.
- Ask about any family history of autoimmune disease such as diabetes, thyroid disease, alopecia. Coeliac disease is commoner in some populations, e.g. the west of Ireland.
- Ask about the onset of symptoms: are they related to the introduction of gluten products in the diet?

Q4: What clinical examination would you perform, and why?

A4

- Plot height and weight on a growth chart.
- Include previous measurements if possible, and see if the child has been crossing centiles downwards.
- Look for signs of wasting, in particular in the buttocks. Look for pallor (anaemia).

 Q5: What investigations would be most helpful, and why?

A5

- Full blood count to look for anaemia. Consider measuring total IgA.
- Check calcium, and alkaline phosphatase for evidence of rickets.
- Blood test for anti-gliadin antibodies, anti-endomysial antibodies, and tissue transglutaminase antibodies. If negative, consider allergy and breath testing.
- If autoantibodies for coeliac disease are present, then a jejunal biopsy should be performed, to look for flattened villi and inflammatory infiltrate.

Q6: What treatment options are appropriate?

A6

Treatment of coeliac disease is by excluding gluten from the diet.

ᴪᴪ OSCE counselling cases

OSCE COUNSELLING CASE 10.1 – My 7-year-old son keeps getting tummy ache on the way to school.

- Recurrent abdominal pain which is sufficient to interrupt normal activities occurs in at least 10 per cent of school-age children.

- Less than 10 per cent of affected children will have a definable organic cause. In 90 per cent the cause is functional abdominal pain.

- Functional abdominal pain is characteristically peri-umbilical, worse on waking, associated with a family history of abdominal pain or migraine, and not accompanied by any other features of ill health.

- It is important that a full history and examination are performed to exclude other causes, such as threadworms or constipation.

- It may be helpful to explain the pain to the child and parent as 'the intestine becoming so sensitive that it is as if the child can feel the food going round the bends'.

- About half of affected children have a rapid resolution of their symptoms, following referral.

- About one-quarter resolve gradually.

- About one-quarter go on to develop irritable bowel syndrome as adults.

- No medical treatment is required.

OSCE COUNSELLING CASE 10.2 – My 10-year-old daughter is constipated, and this is very distressing. Can you give her something?

- Constipation is the infrequent painful passage of hard stools.

- It is common in children, and is sometimes precipitated by a superficial perianal tear.

- Sometimes it is exacerbated by stress, and children may withhold stool for fear of the associated pain. The rectum then becomes full and distended and the sensation of needing to defaecate is lost. Involuntary soiling usually follows as the full rectum overflows.

- Examination may reveal an abdominal mass which is indentable; on rectal examination the stool is palpable down to the anal margin.

- It is important to explain to the child and parents that constipation is common, soiling is involuntary, and recovery of normal bowel habit takes as long as the constipation took to develop.

- Mild cases of constipation may respond to mild laxatives (e.g. lactulose) and extra fluids.

- In more severe cases, treatment begins with stool softeners for 2–3 weeks (e.g. docusate), followed by large doses of powerful oral laxatives (picosulphate or senna) until the stools are liquid. This is followed by regular doses of a stimulant laxative such as senna to prevent reaccumulation of stool.

- Relapse is common, and positive encouragement by the child's family and doctor are essential.

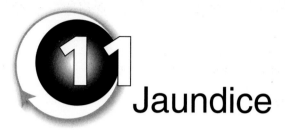

Jaundice

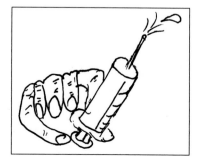

? Questions for each of the clinical cases

Q1: What is the likely differential diagnosis?
Q2: What issues in the given history support the diagnosis?
Q3: What additional features in the history would you seek to support a particular diagnosis?
Q4: What clinical examination would you perform, and why?
Q5: What investigations would be most helpful, and why?
Q6: What treatment options are appropriate?

Clinical cases

● CASE 11.1 – My newborn baby is yellow.

A 3-day-old term baby is noted to be yellow by his mother. He is breast-fed and is making slow progress.

● CASE 11.2 – My 3-week-old baby is still jaundiced.

A 3-week-old girl was noted by the health visitor to have persisting jaundice. She is still breast-fed, but has not yet regained her birth weight.

● CASE 11.3 – My 7-year-old son has developed jaundice.

A 7-year-old boy was referred for investigation of malaise, fever and jaundice. He has dark urine and pale stools.

🏃 OSCE counselling cases

OSCE COUNSELLING CASE 11.1 – Why is my newborn baby yellow?

OSCE COUNSELLING CASE 11.2 – I'm worried that my 3-week-old baby is still jaundiced?

Key concepts

In order to work through the core clinical cases in this chapter, you will need to understand the following key concepts.

Metabolism of bilirubin

- Unconjugated bilirubin is formed following the break-down of erythrocytes, conjugated in the liver by glucuronyl transferase and secreted in bile. In the gut, conjugated bilirubin is further metabolized to urobilinogen (excreted in urine) and stercobilinogen (excreted in faeces). Some is deconjugated and reabsorbed (enterohepatic circulation).

Physiological jaundice

- Common in newborn babies, and occurs usually between 3–7 days of age.
- Precipitating factors include a high postnatal haemoglobin, shorter erythrocyte life span, reduced fluid intake and bruising. In addition, the neonatal liver is less efficient at conjugating bilirubin.
- The serum bilirubin is always >90 per cent unconjugated. This condition is self-limiting, and only requires treatment if the serum bilirubin becomes very high (>300 μmol/L in term babies).

Pathological jaundice

- Any jaundice which is caused by a pathological process.
- In the neonate, it can be subdivided into early (<24 hours) and prolonged (>2 weeks) jaundice. Early jaundice is likely to be due to erythrocyte haemolysis (e.g. Rhesus isoimmunization, ABO incompatibility, spherocytosis). The serum bilirubin is unconjugated.
- A high conjugated component to the serum bilirubin (>15–20%) suggests an obstructive cause (see below).
- Breast milk jaundice is a benign cause of prolonged jaundice. Sepsis may cause jaundice in the newborn. Any baby who is jaundiced and unwell should be considered to have a pathological cause, until proved otherwise.

Obstructive jaundice

- A high conjugated bilirubin, pale stools (lack of stercobilinogen) and dark urine (presence of bilirubin) indicates an obstructive cause which may be either intrahepatic (e.g. hepatitis) or extrahepatic (e.g. biliary atresia).
- The conjugated component of total bilirubin should always be checked in any baby with jaundice at more than 2 weeks of age. A delay in the diagnosis of biliary atresia beyond 6 weeks of age reduces the likelihood of successful surgery for that condition (biliary drainage by a Kasai portoenterostomy).
- It can be difficult to distinguish clinically between neonatal hepatitis and biliary atresia, and a radionucleotide scan (or occasionally a liver biopsy) is usually indicated. Referral to a specialist paediatric hepatology service is advised.

Hepatitis

- Neonatal hepatitis can occur in a wide range of disease processes including congenital infections (e.g. toxoplasmosis, cytomegalovirus (CMV)) and metabolic diseases (e.g. alpha-1-antitrypsin deficiency). In older children, Hepatitis A, B and C, glandular fever and CMV infection can cause acute liver inflammation.

Answers

 CASE 11.1 – My newborn baby is yellow.

 Q1: What is the likely differential diagnosis?

A1

- Physiological jaundice.
- Haemolysis.
- Sepsis.
- Inherited metabolic disorder, e.g. glucose 6-phosphate dehydrogenase (G-6PD) deficiency, galactosaemia.

 Q2: What issues in the given history support the diagnosis?

A2

- The baby is at the age at which physiological jaundice is likely to present.
- Breast feeding may lead to reduced fluid intake initially. Some normal babies are slow to establish breast feeding, but this may indicate lethargy and suggest a pathological process such as sepsis.

Q3: What additional features in the history would you seek to support a particular diagnosis?

A3

- Ask about feeding activity. Does he suck well? Is the baby pyrexial, excessively sleepy or lethargic?
- Has he passed normal urine and stool? Clinical assessment of level of jaundice.
- Check maternal blood group and presence of antenatal antibodies (e.g. anti D).
- Enquire about previous babies or family history of jaundice.

Q4: What clinical examination would you perform, and why?

A4

- Assessment of baby's well-being, check for hepatosplenomegaly and signs of sepsis (lethargy, high-pitched cry, mottling, tense fontanelle).

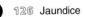 **Q5: What investigations would be most helpful, and why?**

A5

- Serum bilirubin. Unconjugated and conjugated. To define degree of jaundice and exclude significant conjugated component.

- Blood group and direct antibody test (DAT) or Coombs test (evidence of haemolysis due to ABO incompatibility or Rhesus disease).

- Urine for reducing substances (Clinitest), including glucose. To exclude galactosaemia and fructosaemia.

- Urine culture (to exclude urinary tract infection, UTI).

 Q6: What treatment options are appropriate?

A6

- In a well baby with no evidence of haemolysis, the most likely cause is physiological jaundice. If the serum bilirubin is <300 μmol/L, no specific treatment is necessary other than encouraging fluid intake.

- If the bilirubin rises to < 300 μmol/L, then treatment with phototherapy will break down the bilirubin to harmless by-products.

- In haemolytic jaundice the bilirubin may rise rapidly to a level which is potentially dangerous (levels >450 μmol/L may cross the blood–brain barrier and cause kernicterus). Phototherapy may be insufficient in this case, and exchange transfusion may be required.

- If the urine contains reducing substances (not glucose), exclude galactosaemia and fructosaemia.

CASE 11.2 – My 3-week-old baby is still jaundiced.

Q1: What is the likely differential diagnosis?

A1

- Breast milk jaundice.
- Urinary tract infection (UTI).
- Neonatal hepatitis.
- Extrahepatic biliary atresia.

 Q2: What issues in the given history support the diagnosis?

A2

The baby is receiving breast milk and is too old for physiological or haemolytic jaundice. The baby's weight gain is poor, which suggests either inadequate intake or a pathological process.

Q3: What additional features in the history would you seek to support a particular diagnosis?

A3

- Ask about feeding activity and weight gain in more detail.

- Is the baby pyrexial, excessively sleepy or lethargic?

- Enquire about the colour of urine and stool. Is the urine smelly? (a fishy smell may occur with UTI)

- Clinical assessment of level of jaundice.

- Enquire about previous babies or family history of jaundice.

 Q4: What clinical examination would you perform, and why?

A4

General examination, assessment of well-being. Re-check weight, examine for hepatosplenomegaly.

 Q5: What investigations would be most helpful, and why?

A5

- Serum bilirubin. Unconjugated and conjugated. To define degree of jaundice and exclude significant conjugated component.

- If normal conjugated component and normal stools/urine, check urine for reducing substances and culture.

- If high conjugated component, check liver function tests (AST, ALT, γ-GT), TORCH screen (for Toxoplasma, Rubella, Cytomegalovirus, Herpes simplex) α-1- antitrypsin phenotype.

- Radionucleotide excretion scan to assess biliary excretion.

 Q6: What treatment options are appropriate?

A6

- If normal conjugated component and normal stools/urine. Advise regarding breast-feeding and milk intake; re-weigh regularly until thriving.

- Conjugated jaundice – urgent referral to paediatric hepatologist for further assessment and diagnosis.

● Case 11.3 – My 7-year-old son has developed jaundice.

Q1: What is the likely differential diagnosis?

A1

- Viral hepatitis (A, B or C).
- Infectious mononucleosis (glandular fever).
- Cytomegalovirus infection.
- Wilson's disease.
- Chronic active hepatitis.

Q2: What issues in the given history support the diagnosis?

A2

- The combination of jaundice, dark urine and pale stools suggest acute liver inflammation.
- Malaise and fever suggest an infective process.

Q3: What additional features in the history would you seek to support a particular diagnosis?

A3

- Ask about prodromal illness with anorexia, abdominal pain, diarrhoea and vomiting.
- Also ask about sore throat (glandular fever).
- Check recent travel abroad, illness in close contacts and family history.

Q4: What clinical examination would you perform, and why?

A4

- Examine abdomen for tender hepatomegaly ± splenomegaly.
- Examine eyes for Kayser Fleischer rings (Wilson's disease).
- Check for lymph node enlargement (glandular fever).

Q5: What investigations would be most helpful, and why?

A5

- Hepatitis A IgM antibodies: if negative consider:

  - Hepatitis B sAg;

  - Blood film for atypical mononuclear cells and monospot test Epstein–Barr virus IgM antibodies (glandular fever);

  - Cytomegalovirus (CMV) IgM;

  - Serum immunoglobulins and tissue autoantibodies (chronic active hepatitis); and

  - Serum caeruloplasmin and urinary copper (Wilson's disease).

 Q6: What treatment options are appropriate?

A6

- If the diagnosis is hepatitis A or B, glandular fever or CMV infection, then no specific treatment is indicated.

- The rare condition of Wilson's disease may need treatment with penicillamine.

- In hepatitis C or chronic active hepatitis the patient should be referred to a hepatologist.

👥 OSCE counselling cases

OSCE COUNSELLING CASE 11.1 – Why is my newborn baby yellow?

The baby has physiological jaundice. This is a common condition, but it can cause parental anxiety.

● Physiological jaundice is a self-limiting condition. Most babies with this condition do not need treatment, but should be encouraged to drink plenty of fluid. Occasionally, the jaundice level reaches a point which requires intervention, and the most usual treatment is phototherapy (blue light which breaks down bilirubin into harmless metabolites), usually for a day or so.

● The reasons that babies become jaundiced is usually because their blood count (haemoglobin, Hb) is high and Hb is broken down to bilirubin. Newborn babies' blood cells are broken down faster than those of adults, and their livers in the first few days of life cannot metabolize the bilirubin as efficiently. Newborn babies also tend to take less fluid in the first day or so of life, and may have bruises from the delivery. These factors may also contribute to jaundice.

● A simple heel prick blood test will indicate the level of jaundice and the need for treatment. Other simple routine tests may also be performed to exclude other causes of jaundice (e.g. urinalysis, blood group and Coombs' test).

● If the baby is unwell, then the cause of jaundice is unlikely to be physiological and further urgent investigations may be necessary.

OSCE COUNSELLING CASE 11.2 – I'm worried that my 3-week-old baby is still jaundiced?

The baby is well, afebrile and breast feeding well with good weight gain. Examination is normal and the stool and urine are normal colour. The serum bilirubin is all unconjugated.

● The commonest cause for prolonged jaundice is breast milk jaundice. However, there is not a specific test that we can do to confirm this, so we need to consider other important causes. That is why we have asked you about your baby and performed a blood test.

● Bilirubin forms bile which is normally broken down in the intestines, and it is this that make stools a yellow or brown colour. In a very serious condition where the bile cannot get into the intestines, bilirubin builds up in the blood and can pass out in the urine, making it turn dark brown. The combination of pale stools (like putty) and dark urine should alert us that there is a problem. It is important that this condition (biliary atresia) is treated as soon as possible before irreversible damage occurs in the liver. That your baby's stools and urine are normal colour and the blood test shows only one type of bilirubin (unconjugated) is very reassuring.

● Sometimes an infection (particularly of the urine) can cause jaundice. The fact that your baby is well, does not have a fever, is feeding well and thriving makes this unlikely.

● By far the most likely cause is jaundice from breast milk. This is common, harmless and needs no treatment. It usually resolves in 2–3 weeks. The presence of a substance (α-glucuronidase) in the breast milk leads to a slight increase in the absorption of bilirubin back from the intestine (by deconjugating bilirubin in the bowel and increasing enterohepatic circulation).

● There is no need to stop breast feeding to confirm the diagnosis. This will only deprive your baby of the important nutrients and substances which improve immunity that breast milk contains.

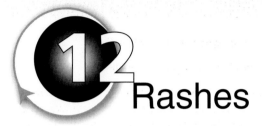

Rashes

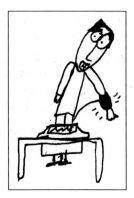

? Questions for each of the clinical cases

Q1: What is the likely differential diagnosis?
Q2: What issues in the given history support the diagnosis?
Q3: What additional features in the history would you seek to support a particular diagnosis?
Q4: What clinical examination would you perform, and why?
Q5: What investigations would be most helpful, and why?
Q6: What treatment options are appropriate?

Clinical cases

● CASE 12.1 – My 6-month-old baby has dry, itchy skin with a red scaly rash.

This baby has always had dry skin, but recently it has become worse and is now red and itchy. There is a family history of asthma and allergies.

● CASE 12.2 – My 18-month-old has bruising over his shins and knees.

This boy – who is otherwise well – has just started climbing upstairs. He is very adventurous, and recently his mother has noticed more bruises on his legs.

● CASE 12.3 – My 5-year-old son has dark red spots on his legs and buttocks.

This boy had a viral illness a few days ago and has not recovered from this. He has a fever and is miserable, but not particularly unwell. Today he has developed dark red spots on his legs and buttocks. These spots do not blanch when pressed.

⚤ OSCE counselling cases

OSCE COUNSELLING CASE 12.1 – **My newborn baby has a red rash in the nappy area.**

OSCE COUNSELLING CASE 12.2 – **I am worried that there has been a case of meningococcal disease at my child's school. Please could you tell me about meningococcal disease and the symptoms, including looking for skin rashes?**

Key concepts

In order to work through the core clinical cases in this chapter, you will need to understand the following key concepts.

- Erythematous rashes are very common in infancy and childhood.

- Most are not serious and resolve spontaneously or with simple treatment.

- Serious infections may also present with rash, and it is important to differentiate between serious and minor illness.

Exanthems

- Exanthems are widespread erythematous rashes which are usually associated with systemic symptoms such as fever, malaise, myalgia and headache.

- They are commonly caused by infectious agents, particularly viruses and occasionally bacteria.

- Exanthems are very common in childhood. Examples include: measles (caused by a paramyxovirus virus), chicken pox (caused by varicella zoster virus), rubella (caused by rubivirus), scarlet fever (caused by streptococcus A), fifth disease (caused by parvovirus B19) and hand, foot and mouth disease (caused by Coxsackie virus A16).

- Exanthems usually have a characteristic appearance to the rash and are associated with a pre-rash prodromal period.

- Some exanthems such as meningococcal disease can be life-threatening and require urgent diagnosis and treatment; other exanthems follow a fairly benign course, but occasionally serious sequelae may develop (e.g. encephalitis following measles).

- Specific immunizations are available against certain exanthems such as measles and rubella.

Other erythematous rashes

- In addition to the exanthems, the commonest erythematous rashes which occur in childhood are eczema, urticaria (or hives), candidiasis, ringworm, impetigo and scabies.

- These conditions usually present with a red itchy rash.

- Eczema is often scaly and may occur on any part of the body, particularly affecting the flexor creases of the elbows and knees.

- Urticaria occurs as a result of an allergic response, and is usually light red in colour with raised edges. It can be very transient, and occurs more commonly on the trunk.

- Candidiasis and ringworm are fungal infections. *Candida* normally affects the groin area, and appears as red plaques. Ringworm can affect any part of the body, and appears as circular plaques.

- Impetigo is a bacterial infection (caused by staphylococcal or streptococcal bacteria); although it can occur on any part of the body, it usually appears around the mouth and nose as a golden crust over a red base.

- Scabies is an intensely itchy rash caused by a mite which burrows under the skin. Commonly occurring on the hands or around the waistline, the rash appears as raised red spots which occasionally crust over.

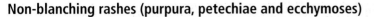

Non-blanching rashes (purpura, petechiae and ecchymoses)

- Purpura are reddish-purple lesions which occur as a result of extravasation of blood into the skin. Petechiae are pin-point-sized purpura, and ecchymoses are >1 cm in size.

- They can be differentiated from erythematous lesions in that they are non-blanching – that is, the lesion does not blanch when pressure is applied to it. (Tumbler test: press a glass onto the lesion to see if it blanches.)

- These rashes can occur in a variety of conditions, including trauma, thrombocytopaenia, vasculitic conditions and meningococcal disease.

- Henoch–Schönlein purpura is an allergic vasculitis of unknown aetiology which affects young children. It typically presents with a low-grade fever and a purpuric rash on the legs and buttocks. It is a self-limiting condition, but can result in more severe complications if haemorrhage occurs in the joints, kidneys or intestine.

- Childhood leukaemia may present with a purpuric rash or ecchymoses as a consequence of thrombocytopaenia.

- The presence of a purpuric rash in an unwell child should always raise concerns about meningococcal disease (see below).

- Ecchymoses for which there is an inadequate explanation of cause, or those with an unusual distribution (e.g. slap marks or finger grip bruises), should always raise suspicion of non-accidental injury (NAI).

Meningococcal disease

- Meningococcal disease is a serious bacterial infection (septicaemia and/or meningitis) with a high morbidity and mortality rate. Unless treated promptly, this condition is invariably fatal.

- It occurs as a result of systemic infection with *Neisseria meningitides* (meningococcus). Thirteen serotypes (strains) of this bacterium exist; strains B and C are the commonest in the UK.

- Symptoms include fever, headache, drowsiness, vomiting and confusion. The presence of any of these symptoms and a purpuric (non-blanching) rash (press a glass against the lesion to confirm this if necessary) warrants urgent medical attention and antibiotic treatment (intramuscular benzylpenicillin if not in hospital).

- A vaccine for meningococcus C is now available, and is given to all infants with diphtheria, tetanus, pertussis, *Haemophilus influenza* B and polio at 2, 3 and 4 months (q.v.).

- Vaccines against some (but not all) of the other serotypes are available.

- Close contacts and people who live in the same house as a case are significantly more likely to develop the disease than non-contacts. Chemoprophylaxis (antibiotics to prevent the disease occurring; rifampicin in children and ciprofloxacin in adults) should be given to all significant contacts, and then immunization (if the specific vaccine is available for the serotype causing the disease).

Answers

 CASE 12.1 – My 6-month-old baby has dry, itchy skin with a red scaly rash.

 Q1: What is the likely differential diagnosis?

A1

- Infantile eczema (atopic dermatitis).
- Scabies.
- Fungal infection (candidiasis or ringworm).

Q2: What issues in the given history support the diagnosis?

A2

- Dry skin would suggest eczema.
- The strong family history of atopy (asthma and allergy) would also fit with this diagnosis.

 Q3: What additional features in the history would you seek to support a particular diagnosis?

A3

- Confirm family history of allergy; ask about eczema in infancy in close family members.
- Ask about localization of the rash (e.g. on face, trunk and in flexural creases).
- Any other evidence of atopy, e.g. wheezing. Has there been a preceding prodrome and symptomatology suggestive of an exanthem?

Q4: What clinical examination would you perform, and why?

A4

- Examine the skin over the whole body. Is there dry skin and erythema over most of the trunk face and limbs, particularly creases? Is it dry, or is it moist and weeping (suggesting infected eczema)? Is it localized to the nappy area, and are the lesions well-circumscribed (suggestive of fungal infection)? Are the lesions raised and localized to the fingers, wrists and groin (suggestive of scabies)?
- Examine the chest for hyperinflation, Harrison's sulci, sternal bowing and wheezes.

Q5: What investigations would be most helpful, and why?

A5

- Specific investigations are not necessary if eczema is the most likely clinical diagnosis.
- Skin scrapings from a suspected fungal lesion should be sent for mycology.
- Scabies can be confirmed by extracting the mite from the skin burrows and examining it under a microscope.

 Q6: What treatment options are appropriate?

A6

- Eczema is treated in the first instance with regular, liberal application of emollients and use of bath oil instead of soap.
- More severe exacerbations will respond to sparing application of topical mild steroid ointment (e.g. 0.5–1% hydrocortisone) in short courses (no more than 2 weeks at a time).
- Fungal infections respond well to antifungal creams (see below). Scabies is treated with permethrin; the whole family require treatment to prevent reinfection.

CASE 12.2 – My 18-month-old has bruising over his shins and knees.

 Q1: What is the likely differential diagnosis?

A1

- Normal toddler bruising.
- Non-accidental injury (NAI).
- Henoch–Schönlein purpura (HSP).
- Clotting disorder (e.g. idiopathic thrombocytopaenic purpura, haemophilia).
- Leukaemia (or other conditions causing thrombocytopaenia).

 Q2: What issues in the given history support the diagnosis?

A2

- At 18 months of age children will be toddling, but may have frequent falls as they are learning. Active adventurous children are more likely to tumble and acquire minor bruising as a consequence.

Q3: What additional features in the history would you seek to support a particular diagnosis?

A3

Enquire about the following:

- Walking activity and frequency of falls.

- Painful swollen joints (haemarthroses) which occur in coagulation disorders (e.g. haemophilia).

- Abdominal pain, painful joints, preceding coryzal illness (e.g. as in HSP).

- Lethargy, pallor, mucosal bleeding or other features of ill health (e.g. as in leukaemia).

- Take a social history and enquire about carers and family dynamics.

- Does the history fit the pattern of bruising observed, and was appropriate medical attention sought? Are the histories of different care-givers consistent (if suspicious of NAI).

 Q4: What clinical examination would you perform, and why?

A4

- Examine all the skin for bruising and or petechiae. Are they extensive or large? Is the bruising localized to the lower limbs (suggesting accidental bruising or HSP; bruising in HSP tends to be localized to the extensor surfaces of the lower limbs and buttocks) or generalized and/or associated with mucosal bleeding (suggesting a coagulopathy or leukaemia).

- Are the joints swollen or tender?

- Are there any suspicious lesions which might suggest NAI? (e.g. slap or grip marks, burns or weals, suspected fractures).

- Check for lymphadenopathy, hepatosplenomegaly (suggestive of leukaemia).

Q5: What investigations would be most helpful, and why?

A5

If the child is well, the bruises are small and localized to parts of the body involved with falls (shins, knees occasionally head), the explanation is appropriate, and there are no other abnormal findings on examination, then no further investigation is warranted.

However, if the bruising is excessive, widespread, associated with trivial accidents, swollen joints, pallor or systemic signs of ill health, it would be appropriate to perform the following initial investigations:

- Full blood count (FBC, haemoglobin, white blood cell and platelet count) and blood film.

- Coagulation screen (prothrombin time, partial thromboplastin time).

- Consider bone marrow check if FBC abnormal.

- If in doubt, consider checking whether child is on the child protection register and whether the GP and health visitor have any concerns, and discussing with a paediatrician. If there are concerns about NAI, then the child protection process should be initiated. This should involve a senior doctor and social services.

 Q6: What treatment options are appropriate?

A6

Toddler bruising requires no treatment.

 CASE 12.3 – My 5-year-old son has dark red spots on his legs and buttocks.

 Q1: What is the likely differential diagnosis?

A1

- Henoch–Schönlein purpura (HSP or anaphylactoid purpura).
- Meningococcal disease.
- Idiopathic thrombocytopaenic purpura (ITP).

 Q2: What issues in the given history support the diagnosis?

A2

The localization of the purpuric rash to the legs and buttocks, and the preceding viral illness would suggest HSP.

Q3: What additional features in the history would you seek to support a particular diagnosis?

A3

- Enquire about fever, joint pain or swelling, abdominal pain and haematuria (these symptoms may be associated with HSP).
- Ask about photophobia, headache, neck stiffness and lethargy (which may be associated with meningococcal disease).

Q4: What clinical examination would you perform, and why?

A4

- Assess overall well-being. Are there features of serious illness?
- Confirm that the rash is non-blanching. Examine joints and abdomen.

Q5: **What investigations would be most helpful, and why?**

A5

- Check urine for blood and protein. Also, check blood pressure (25–50% of patients with HSP will have renal involvement, and a small proportion will develop renal impairment).

- Check stool for occult blood if significant abdominal pain (haemorrhage into the gut can occur and may occasionally cause intussusception).

- Check platelet count and coagulation – to exclude ITP and other coagulopathies.

- If doubt about diagnosis, perform a blood culture.

Q6: **What treatment options are appropriate?**

A6

HSP is usually self-limiting, and no treatment is required for except analgesia for joint pain. If complications occur (e.g. renal or gut involvement), then supportive therapy may be necessary.

ᴬᴬ OSCE counselling cases

OSCE COUNSELLING CASE 12.1 – My newborn baby has a red rash in the nappy area.

- Nappy rash usually occurs as a result of contact dermatitis (ammonia from urine) or fungal infection (candida or thrush). Occasionally, bacterial infection (e.g. staphylococcal) may occur.

- Dermatitis usually presents as a widespread groin rash which spares the creases.

- *Candida* usually appears as red plaques with occasional smaller spots (satellite lesions), and the creases are involved. Sometimes, *Candida* can appear in the mouth as white plaques on the inner cheek or tongue.

- Nappy rash is very common, and not usually due to parental neglect.

- Cleaning the area with water and cotton wool may be less irritant than disposable 'baby wipes' (which may contain alcohol or detergent).

- Treatment of dermatitis involves barrier creams such as zinc oxide and exposure to the air (whenever possible).

- *Candida* responds to antifungal creams (e.g. miconazole, nystatin). The groin and the mouth may both need treatment.

OSCE COUNSELLING CASE 12.2 – I am worried that there has been a case of meningococcal disease at my child's school. Please could you tell me about meningococcal disease and the symptoms, including looking for skin rashes?

- Meningococcal disease is a serious infection caused by certain bacteria which may cause blood poisoning (septicaemia) or inflammation of the lining of the brain and spinal cord (meningitis).

- *Neisseria meningitidis* (meningococci) is the bacterium responsible. It is found in the noses and throats of 5–10 per cent of the population, but rarely causes serious disease unless it enters the bloodstream or spinal fluid.

- Meningococci can spread among people through the exchange of saliva and other respiratory secretions during activities such as coughing and kissing, but they are not as contagious as the common cold or influenza. They are not spread by simply breathing the same air as a person with meningococcal disease.

- Common symptoms of meningococcal disease include high temperature, headache, drowsiness and vomiting. A stiff neck can occur with the meningitis, and an unusual rash occurs with the septicaemia. Typically, this rash is dark red and does not blanch when pressure is applied. Use a glass to see if the rash blanches when pressed.

- If these symptoms occur – or if you are in any doubt at all – it is very important that medical advice is sought urgently, because if the disease has developed it is very important to administer antibiotics straight away. These should be given directly into a vein or a muscle, and not by mouth.

- There are 13 different types (strains) of the meningococcus, and vaccines are available against some, but not all, of them. One is now given routinely with the other childhood vaccines.

- Close contacts and people in the same house as a person who has the disease are more at risk of developing it themselves. In this situation, antibiotics should be given to prevent this occurring (antibiotic prophylaxis). These antibiotics can be taken by mouth, and do not need to be given into a vein or muscle.

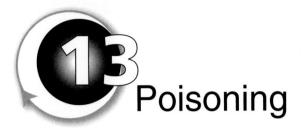

Poisoning

Questions

Clinical cases

Key concepts

Answers

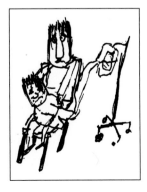

? **Questions for each of the clinical cases**

Q1: What is the likely differential diagnosis?
Q2: What issues in the given history support the diagnosis?
Q3: What additional features in the history would you seek to support a particular diagnosis?
Q4: What clinical examination would you perform, and why?
Q5: What investigations would be most helpful, and why?
Q6: What treatment options are appropriate?

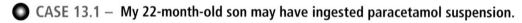

Clinical cases

● CASE 13.1 – My 22-month-old son may have ingested paracetamol suspension.

A 22-month-old boy has been drinking from an open bottle of paracetamol suspension. The bottle was previously half full, and is now nearly empty.

● CASE 13.2 – My 4-year-old daughter has mistaken iron tablets for sweets, and has eaten some.

A 4-year-old and her friends have mistaken iron tablets for sweets, and eaten a number of them. The mother is uncertain how many were in the bottle, but there are quite a few left.

● CASE 13.3 – My 11-year-old son is complaining of headaches, confusion, nausea and vomiting and shortness of breath.

An 11-year-old boy presents with headaches, nausea and vomiting, confusion and shortness of breath. The symptoms have been getting worse, but resolved during a few days' stay with his cousins. He is worse in the mornings, but improves when at school.

♟ OSCE counselling cases

OSCE COUNSELLING CASE 13.1 – My toddler has ingested washing powder. What will happen to him, and how can I prevent this happening again?

OSCE COUNSELLING CASE 13.2 – My 14-year-old daughter has deliberately taken a paracetamol overdose. What treatment does she need?

🔑 Key concepts

In order to work through the core clinical cases in this chapter, you will need to understand the following key concepts.

- The ingestion of a potentially toxic substance is relatively common, and can occur either deliberately or accidentally.

- The majority of children will be asymptomatic following ingestion and require no specific treatment.

- A careful history is essential, paying particular attention to the precise nature and dose of the substance ingested. An assessment of the potential maximum dose ingested should be made.

- A careful examination, including full neurological assessment is also essential.

- When treatments are necessary they usually involve delay in absorption or augmentation of excretion. Examples of such treatments include activated charcoal, whole-bowel irrigation (e.g. in iron ingestion), haemofiltration/haemodialysis (some drugs, e.g. theophylline, carbamazepine) and alkaline diuresis (salicylate ingestion).

- Supportive management including airway maintenance and treatment of the following is occasionally required in serious poisoning: dehydration and shock, acidosis, hypoglycaemia and convulsions.

- Many commonly ingested substances are relatively harmless and require no specific investigation or treatment; these include oral contraceptives, silica gel, vitamin tablets (without iron), antibiotics, cosmetics, paints, washing powder.

- Some commonly ingested substances have a high toxicity; these include iron tablets, dishwasher powder, toilet cistern blocks and antihistamines.

- Some poisons have specific antidotes, e.g. N-acetylcysteine for paracetamol, naloxone for opiates, and desferrioxamine for iron.

- If there are any doubts about the management, the local poisons unit should be contacted promptly.

Answers

 ● CASE 13.1 – **My 22-month-old son may have ingested paracetamol suspension.**

 Q1: What is the likely differential diagnosis?

A1

- Possible paracetamol ingestion.

- Normal child (i.e. no ingestion).

 Q2: What issues in the given history support the diagnosis?

A2

The child has been found with the bottle, and the contents are reduced.

 Q3: What additional features in the history would you seek to support a particular diagnosis?

A3

- Find out exactly how much was in the bottle, and what dose per mL of paracetamol is contained in the suspension. Establish the maximum possible dose ingested.

- Establish as precisely as possible the timing of the ingestion.

- Was there any evidence of spillage? For example, on the floor or on the clothes.

- Was anyone else with him at the time?

- Has he vomited since being found?

 Q4: What clinical examination would you perform, and why?

A4

- Check his body weight (so that the maximum dose per kilogram can be established).

Q5: What investigations would be most helpful, and why?

A5

- It is unlikely that a significant quantity of paracetamol will have been ingested. Paracetamol suspension is usually 24 mg/mL, but a stronger preparation of 48 mg/mL is available. Significant paracetamol ingestion is much more likely with tablets (usually 500 mg per tablet). However, given the uncertainty it would be prudent to measure the serum paracetamol level (as described below) in this case.

- In all cases, if it is possible that more than 150 mg/kg has been ingested, a venous blood sample for serum paracetamol level should be taken 4 hours after ingestion. (It is important that the level is not measured before this time, as interpretation is very difficult.)

- Plot the blood result against time after ingestion treatment action chart.

- If greater than 150 mg/kg has been ingested more than 8 hours previously, do not wait for a serum level before starting treatment. (It is also important to remember that paracetamol poisoning does not cause symptoms in the early stages, and a delay in treatment may be fatal.) If a child has also drunk alcohol or is taking anticonvulsants, this increases the risk of hepatotoxicity, and therefore a lower threshold for treatment is warranted.

- Paracetamol is hepatotoxic, and therefore clotting (INR), creatinine and alanine transferase levels should also be checked. Peak hepatotoxicity occurs at 72–96 hours post-ingestion.

 Q6: What treatment options are appropriate?

A6

- Toxic levels of paracetamol are treated with *N*-acetylcysteine.

- If the amount ingested is not greater than 150 mg/kg, then no treatment is required.

- The parents should be advised about safe storage of medicines and other potentially harmful substances, and the health visitor and GP should be informed so that they can reinforce safety in the home through child health surveillance.

CASE 13.2 – My 4-year-old daughter has mistaken iron tablets for sweets, and has eaten some.

 Q1: What is the likely differential diagnosis?

A1

- Iron toxicity.

- Potential iron toxicity in the child's friends.

Q2: What issues in the given history support the diagnosis?

A2

The child has been playing with friends, but it is unclear how many tablets there were to start with, or how many were ingested. It is therefore possible that none or all of the children may have ingested a potentially toxic amount of iron. In view of this, the only safe option is to assume that they all may have ingested a significant quantity.

Q3: What additional features in the history would you seek to support a particular diagnosis?

A3

- Find out about the specific iron compound and the iron content of each tablet (this is vital, as the amount of elemental iron per tablet varies with the type of preparation).

- Find out about the maximum number of tablets in a full bottle, and how many are left. Were any found on the floor, or in the children's clothing?

- Have any of the children vomited since the ingestion?

- Have any of the children had any other symptoms which may suggest iron toxicity, e.g. diarrhoea, abdominal pain or haematemesis? In severe cases there may be drowsiness, convulsions, metabolic acidosis, shock and multi-organ failure.

 ### Q4: What clinical examination would you perform, and why?

A4

- Check the body weight of each child (so maximum dose per kilogram can be established). The minimum toxic dose of iron in children is estimated to be anywhere from 20 to 60 mg/kg. Fatal poisonings have rarely been reported with less than 60 mg/kg elemental Fe.

- Pulse, respiratory rate and blood pressure.

- Full examination, paying particular attention to the gastrointestinal tract and for evidence of central nervous system depression.

Q5: What investigations would be most helpful, and why?

A5

If there is a risk of toxicity from iron ingestion, the following investigations should be performed in all children:

- Full blood count.

- Serum iron level.

- Plasma electrolytes, including chloride and bicarbonate (for anion gap).

- Blood glucose.

- Plain abdominal X-ray (may show evidence of radio-opaque pills or pill fragments in the gastrointestinal tract).

 ### Q6: What treatment options are appropriate?

A6

Symptomatic and general supportive treatment is vital, with close monitoring of vital signs and aggressive intravenous fluid resuscitation.

- Patients who present early may benefit from whole-bowel irrigation using an osmotically balanced polyethylene glycol-electrolyte solution (this forces the unabsorbed iron through the gastrointestinal tract quickly and helps prevent further absorption of iron).

- Severely affected patients may benefit from the use of intravenous desferrioxamine; this chelates iron, allowing it to be renally excreted.

● CASE 13.3 – My 11-year-old son is complaining of headaches, confusion, nausea and vomiting and shortness of breath.

Q1: What is the likely differential diagnosis?

A1

- Viral illness (e.g. influenza or gastroenteritis).
- Intracranial space-occupying lesion.
- Carbon monoxide poisoning.

Q2: What issues in the given history support the diagnosis?

A2

The chronic nature of the illness with improvement when out of the house should raise the suspicion of carbon monoxide (CO) poisoning. The symptoms of CO poisoning are often vague, and a high degree of suspicion is required.

Q3: What additional features in the history would you seek to support a particular diagnosis?

A3

Enquire about the following:

- The heating system in the house – does it use gas, oil, coal or wood. Also, fuels used in boilers, engines, oil burners, gas fires, water heaters, solid fuel appliances and open fires.

- The colour of the flame from gas appliances (may be yellow rather than blue if ventilation is inadequate), and servicing of equipment and ventilation in the house, particularly in the boy's room.

- If any other members of the family have similar symptoms.

Q4: What clinical examination would you perform, and why?

A4

The consequences of CO poisoning are related to damage from hypoxia and direct CO-mediated damage at a cellular level. The heart and brain are particularly susceptible. The following should therefore be checked:

- Pulse and respiratory rate (may be increased in CO poisoning).

- Blood pressure (may be reduced).

- Check for cyanosis. Oxygen saturations may be unreliable in CO poisoning.

- Full assessment of the central nervous system – looking particularly for hyper-reflexia, incoordination, and visual, hearing or sensory impairment.

 Q5: What investigations would be most helpful, and why?

A5

- Measure carboxyhaemoglobin (COHb) levels (a co-oximeter determines spectrophotometrically the percentage of CO-saturated haemoglobin).

- Check acid–base status and arterial blood gases if severe poisoning is suspected.

- Creatinine kinase levels may indicate the degree of rhabdomyolysis in severe cases.

 Q6: What treatment options are appropriate?

A6

- Immediate treatment with 100 per cent oxygen.

- Supportive therapy (e.g. fluids ± inotropic support, control of seizures, correction of acidosis, etc.).

- Hyperbaric oxygen therapy should be considered in severe cases. Expert advice should be sought in these circumstances.

🏃 OSCE counselling cases

OSCE COUNSELLING CASE 13.1 – My toddler has ingested washing powder. What will happen to him, and how can I prevent this happening again?

- Ingestions of household substances are very common, particularly in the 1- to 4-year age group.

- The risk of serious consequences as a result of ingesting washing powder are low, and no hospital admission or specific treatment is required.

- However, some household substances are potentially very toxic, and it is important to be aware of this. These substances include dishwasher powder, liquids or tablets, oven cleaners, button batteries and toilet cistern blocks, all of which are very corrosive.

- Prevention of ingestion of harmful substances is very important in homes with young children. All potentially poisonous substances should be kept in tamper-proof containers, preferably in a high or locked cupboard.

- Do not store products in anything other than their original container.

- Adequate adult supervision at all times is also required.

OSCE COUNSELLING CASE 13.2 – My 14-year-old daughter has deliberately taken a paracetamol overdose. What treatment does she need?

- Initial treatment of deliberate paracetamol ingestion should be the same as accidental ingestion (q.v.), although the likelihood of paracetamol toxicity is much greater.

- The risk from paracetamol overdose occurs as a result of hepatotoxicity (liver damage).

- If a significant quantity has been ingested, then treatment with intravenous N-acetylcysteine is warranted.

- Deliberate poison ingestion is a common presentation in older children, and can often be in response to precipitating factor (such as an argument with parent or friend) which may appear minor to adults. However, it is important that these events are taken seriously, and not trivialized.

- Individuals who attempt to self harm have a much greater risk of psychiatric illness, and are therefore at risk of repeating the attempt.

- In view of this, all patients taking a deliberate overdose should undergo social, psychological and/or psychiatric assessment prior to discharge.

- This assessment can offer an opportunity for difficulties between adolescents and parents to be discussed.

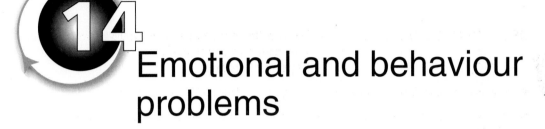

Emotional and behaviour problems

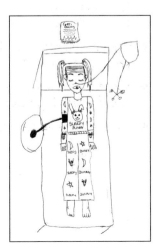

Q1: What is the likely differential diagnosis?
Q2: What issues in the given history support the diagnosis?
Q3: What additional features in the history would you seek to support a particular diagnosis?
Q4: What clinical examination would you perform, and why?
Q5: What investigations would be most helpful, and why?
Q6: What treatment options are appropriate?

Clinical cases

● CASE 14.1 – My 2-year-old girl refuses to eat, won't go to sleep at night, and hits other children.

A 2-year-old girl presents with a history of difficult behaviour since the age of 8 months. She hits other children if they refuse to share their toys with her. She wakes frequently at night, and will not settle unless taken into her parents' bed. She refuses to eat at family meals, preferring to snack on chocolate, crisps and biscuits. The family are asylum seekers, and their neighbours in a council property have been complaining about the noise that the little girl makes. However, the local playgroup have told the health visitor that she is a sociable little girl who interacts well with her peer group.

● CASE 14.2 – My 6-year-old boy is disruptive in class, has no friends, and is aggressive.

A 6-year-old boy has a long history of poor concentration and being disruptive in class, and has difficulty in forming peer relationships. He is aggressive and his school progress is poor.

● CASE 14.3 – My 2-year-old boy doesn't play with other children, isn't speaking, and seems to be in a world of his own.

A 2-year-old boy has a long history of concerns over communication. He has never babbled or spoken intelligible words. He plays alone, and is aggressive if his routines are disturbed.

OSCE counselling cases

OSCE COUNSELLING CASE 14.1 – **My 9-year-old boy wets the bed.**

OSCE COUNSELLING CASE 14.2 – **My 2-year-old boy has nocturnal screaming episodes.**

🔑 Key concepts

In order to work through the core clinical cases in this chapter, you will need to understand the following key concepts.

● Emotional and behavioural problems are common in children and young people. Up to 2 million under-16-year-olds in England may require help from health services at some time, of whom about half have definable mental health disorders, and a smaller number have severe mental illness.

● Children's behaviour and emotional responses are the result of genetic predisposition and environment, of which the family is the major factor.

Attention deficit hyperactivity disorder (ADHD).

ADHD is distinguished from the normal but very active child by three key features:

● Inattention (poor concentration with an inability to maintain attention without distraction): easily distracted, easily moves from one incomplete task to the next, difficulty in following instructions.

● Hyperactivity (difficulty in controlling the amount of physical activity appropriate to the situation): difficult to sit quietly, can talk excessively, fidgets.

● Impulsivity (lacks appropriate forethought): interrupts, difficult in turn-taking.

Hearing, vision and learning problems may also coexist with hyperactivity.

Definitive diagnosis is a specialist task for a neurodevelopmental paediatrician, or a child and adolescent mental health multidisciplinary team.

Pervasive developmental disorder (autism)

The following triad of features that affect function in all situations suggests a pervasive developmental disorder:

● Impairment of reciprocal social interactions (playing alone, failing to make eye contact, doesn't comes for comfort when hurt or upset).

● Impairment of reciprocal communication (has never babbled or spoken intelligible words).

● Restricted range of interests and activities (has marked routines or rituals, which produce violent temper tantrums if disrupted).

Autism may be associated with cognitive impairment, unusual motor features (e.g. flapping hands, walking on tiptoe), general learning disability, fears, phobias, sleeping and eating disturbance, tantrums, self-injury and abnormal sensory responses (e.g. highly sensitive to noise).

Once again, definitive diagnosis is a specialist task for a neurodevelopmental paediatrician or a child and adolescent mental health multidisciplinary team

Complex and often multiple mental and physical health issues need specialist intervention.

Answers

 CASE 14.1 – **My 2-year-old girl refuses to eat, won't go to sleep at night, and hits other children.**

 Q1: **What is the likely differential diagnosis?**

A1

- Preschool behaviour problem.

- Disordered social background.

- Hearing or visual problem.

- Learning problem.

- Hyperactivity.

- Physical or sexual abuse.

 Q2: **What issues in the given history support the diagnosis?**

A2

Tantrums, waking at night and meal refusal are common behavioural problems in the preschool years, and seem likely here in the light of good behaviour in other settings.

 Q3: **What additional features in the history would you seek to support a particular diagnosis?**

A3

- A full developmental history is needed to screen for hearing, vision and learning problems.

- An account of what happens before and at mealtimes, bedtime and playtime is needed, together with a description of the family's responses to the child's behaviour.

- What are the family's main concerns – lack of food/sleep or lack of discipline? In hyperactivity, the child is overactive most of the time, and this seems unlikely here.

Q4: **What clinical examination would you perform, and why?**

A4

- A full physical examination is required, with a particular emphasis on the developmental assessment. An ear, nose and throat examination should be made for signs of visual, hearing or learning problems.

- The child's behaviour in the consulting room can be informative.
- Height and weight should be plotted on a growth chart, in view of the history of meal refusal.

 Q5: What investigations would be most helpful, and why?

A5

- Investigations may not be required.
- A hearing or vision test, or a detailed formal interdisciplinary assessment in the family home or in a child development centre, may be indicated by the history and examination.

Q6: What treatment options are appropriate?

A6

- Reassurance that the child does not have a major organic or mental health disorder, with empathy for the family's plight, is required.
- The family needs advice and encouragement from the doctor, health visitor, social worker and playgroup in order to adopt parenting strategies to modify the child's behaviour.
- Avoid confrontation at mealtimes, bedtime and playtime through avoidance of known antecedents to behaviour; use distraction when confrontations arise.
- Develop a relaxed routine for regular mealtimes and bedtime at the same time each night. Have meals, bathtime and bedtime with other children.
- Use favourite foods and toys as rewards.
- Time out for difficult behaviour, e.g., walk away (return when the child quietens down), separate from other children, remove from family meal, put in a 'naughty corner' for a few minutes.

CASE 14.2 – My 6-year-old boy is disruptive in class, has no friends, and is aggressive.

 Q1: What is the likely differential diagnosis?

A1

- Attention deficit hyperactivity disorder (ADHD).
- Normal, but very active, child.
- Hearing or visual problem.
- Specific learning disability.
- Autistic spectrum disorder.

Q2: What issues in the given history support the diagnosis?

A2

- Poor concentration and disruptive behaviour suggest ADHD, but may also be seen in normal active children.

 Q3: What additional features in the history would you seek to support a particular diagnosis?

A3

- Ask about inattention and degree of physical activity, excessive fidgeting and talking. Is he easily distracted? Can he follow instructions? Ask about social skills, e.g. turn-taking

- A detailed history of relevant risk factors includes details of a family history of hyperactivity, diet, social adversity, and early childhood stresses such as abuse or hospitalization is also needed.

 Q4: What clinical examination would you perform, and why?

A4

- A full physical examination is required, including a neurodevelopmental assessment and ear nose and throat examination.

 Q5: What investigations would be most helpful, and why?

A5

- Consider referral to a specialist team.

Q6: What treatment options are appropriate?

A6

- With ADHD, interprofessional work with parents, teachers and the child is required to build concentration skills, enhance self-esteem, modify extreme behaviour through consistency and clarity of approach.

- In selected cases, medication such as methylphenidate has its place as part of a multiprofessional behaviour programme.

● **CASE 14.3 – My 2-year-old boy doesn't play with other children, isn't speaking, and seems to be in a world of his own.**

 Q1: What is the likely differential diagnosis?

A1

- Pervasive developmental disorder (autism).

- Hearing or visual impairment.

- Learning disability.

- Physical or sexual abuse.

 Q2: What issues in the given history support the diagnosis?

A2

- Poor communication, failure to mix with other children and development of routines are suggestive of autism.

 Q3: What additional features in the history would you seek to support a particular diagnosis?

A3

- A full history is required. Ask about social interactions: eye contact, comfort-seeking, etc. Explore routines and ritual behaviour in more detail.

 Q4: What clinical examination would you perform, and why?

A4

- A full physical examination is required as well as a comprehensive neurodevelopment assessment, mental state examination and an assessment of cognitive function.

 Q5: What investigations would be most helpful, and why?

A5

- Consider referral to a specialist task for a neurodevelopmental paediatrician or a child and adolescent mental health multidisciplinary team.

Q6: What treatment options are appropriate?

A6

- Specific interventions in all developmental disorders are aimed at enabling the young person to achieve their potential, and supporting the family with a community-based multidisciplinary team.

- Intervention to meet a child's emotional, social and educational needs, including the provision of special education.

👥 OSCE counselling cases

OSCE COUNSELLING CASE 14.1 – **My 9-year-old boy wets the bed.**

It seems that this boy has always wet his bed at night. His bowel habit is normal, and he is otherwise in good health. His father wet the bed until he was quite old. The physical examination, including abdominal, spine, lower limb neurology and urinalysis, is normal.

Many treatments have been tried for bedwetting; no single treatment will cure all children, so the important thing is to choose the right thing for each child. The consultation should identify both the child's and the parents' concerns and objectives, and establish a way forward that is acceptable to all.

Facts to remember:

● Bedwetting is common at this age; 3 per cent of normal 10-year-olds wet the bed once a week, or more.

● There is often a family history of bedwetting.

● Usually, children who wet the bed do not have physical or emotional problems.

● Bedwetting can become a problem for many children and their families, particularly once children go to junior school.

What causes bedwetting?

● Bedwetting happens during a type of sleep in which sleep-walking and sleep-talking occur in younger children. The cause is unknown.

● Restricting drinks in the evening does not prevent the episode from occurring.

● Because it happens during sleep, the child has no conscious control over it, so the problem is neither the child's nor the parents' fault.

What can parents do to help?

● Reassure your child, especially if they are upset. You need to be patient and understanding, even though you may feel angry.

● Encourage a good night's sleep. Waking your child to go to the toilet during the night will not help solve the problem.

● Try absorbent pads. The pads go under the bottom sheet to keep the bed drier and more comfortable.

● Encourage your son to shower before he goes to school. The smell of urine is very strong and can hang around. This may make your child feel embarrassed and lead to other problems, such as teasing and name-calling at school.

What treatment may help?

● Your local bedwetting clinic can supply or recommend a bedwetting alarm which wakes the child in the night when he starts wetting. When a child begins to urinate, a sensor (either a bed pad or one worn inside pyjamas) is moistened, and the alarm is triggered. Alarms work best with the professional help of a bedwetting nurse. Alarms need lots of time and commitment on the part of both parents and child to work! About half of all children who complete an alarm programme remain dry after the programme is completed.

● Alarms may be used in conjunction with a suitable reward systems (e.g. star charts) in which the child might receive a star for every dry night, and a reward after a preset number of stars have been earned.

- Certain medications may help, but the problem often occurs again when the medications finish. Thus, medication is most useful for specific events such as nights away from home. All drugs have some side effects.

- Most children grow out of the problem, even without treatment.

OSCE COUNSELLING CASE 14.2 – My 2-year-old boy has nocturnal screaming episodes.

This boy goes to bed without problems but wakes 2 hours later, screaming. The parents find him sitting up in bed, eyes open, disorientated, confused and distressed, but unresponsive to them. He settles back to sleep after a few minutes, and shows no evidence of recall of the episode in the morning. Development and growth history are normal, and physical examination reveals no abnormal signs.

- The history is typical of night terrors.

- This is good news; they do not harm the child in any way, do not signify serious underlying problems, and do not interfere with growth or development. Despite the child's appearance they are not really distressed, i.e. night terrors are not the same as nightmares.

- A night terror is a disturbance of sleep pattern, where very rapid emergence from the first stage of sleep produces a state of high arousal.

- Sleep-walking is a similar phenomenon.

- The child needs reassurance alone.

- The problem settles with time.

- Sometimes, waking the child 15 minutes before the phenomenon usually starts, each night for a week, can cure the problem.

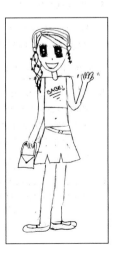

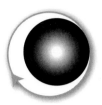

Index